KU-680-097

The Effective Prevention and Management of Post-operative Nausea and Vomiting

Second edition

The Library, Education Centre
Royal Surrey County Hospital
Egerton Road, Guildford, GU2 7XX
Tel: 01483 464137

Class number   WO 184

Computer number H0606285

The Effective Prevention and Management of Post-operative Nausea and Vomiting

Second edition

Edited by

Leo Strunin MD FRCA FRCPC
*Immediate Past President, Association of Anaesthetists, and Past President,
The Royal College of Anaesthetists, London*

David Rowbotham MD MRCP FRCA
*Professor of Anaesthesia and Pain Management, University of Leicester at
Leicester Royal Infirmary*

Andrew Miles MSc MPhil PhD
*Professor of Public Health Sciences and Editor-in-Chief, Journal of Evaluation in Clinical
Practice, Barts and The London, Queen Mary's School of Medicine and Dentistry,
University of London, UK*

Barts and The London
Queen Mary's School of
Medicine and Dentistry

Association of
Anaesthetists of Great
Britain and Ireland

The Royal College
of
Anaesthetists

AESCULAPIUS MEDICAL PRESS
LONDON SAN FRANCISCO SYDNEY

Published by

Aesculapius Medical Press (London, San Francisco, Sydney)
PO Box LB48, London EC1A 1LB, UK

© Aesculapius Medical Press 2003

First published 2003

All rights reserved. No part of this publication may be reproduced or transmitted in any
form or by any means, electronically or mechanically, including photocopying, recording
or any other information storage or retrieval system, without the prior permission in
writing from the publishers.

British Library Cataloguing in Publication Data
A CIP catalogue record for this book is available from the British Library

ISBN: 1 903044 36 7

While the advice and information in this book are believed to be true and accurate at the
time of going to press, neither the authors nor the publishers nor the sponsoring institutions
can accept any legal responsibility or liability for errors or omissions that may be made.
In particular (but without limiting the generality of the preceding disclaimer) every effort
has been made to check drug usages; however, it is possible that errors have been missed.
Furthermore, dosage schedules are constantly being revised and new side effects recognised.
For these reasons, the reader is strongly urged to consult the drug companies' printed
instructions before administering any of the drugs recommended in this book.

Further copies of this volume are available from:

Claudio Melchiorri
Aesculapius Medical Press
PO Box LB48, London EC1A 1LB, UK

Fax: 020 8525 8661
Email: claudio@keyadvances4.demon.co.uk

Copy edited by The Clyvedon Press Ltd, Cardiff, UK

Typeset, printed and bound in Britain
Peter Powell Origination & Print Limited

Contents

Part 4 Ongoing research in PONV

Contributors

Paul L.R. Andrews PhD, Professor of Comparative Physiology, St George's Hospital Medical School, London

Imad T. Awad FCARCSI, Clinical Research Fellow in Pain Management, University of Leicester at Leicester Royal Infirmary

Michael Harmer MD FRCA, Professor of Anaesthesia, University of Wales College of Medicine, and Editor-in-Chief, *Anaesthesia*

Gregg Hobbs FRCA, Consultant in Anaesthesia and Pain Management, Queen's Medical Centre, University Hospital, Nottingham

Philip M. Hopkins MB BS MD FRCA, Professor of Anaesthesia, University of Leeds at St James's University Hospital, Leeds

Philip Howard BPharm MRPharmS, Clinical Pharmacy Manager, St James's University Hospital, Leeds

Roger D. Knaggs PhD MPharmS, Senior Pharmacist, Anaesthesia and Pain Management, Queen's Medical Centre, University Hospital, Nottingham

David J. Rowbotham MD MRCP FRCA, Professor of Anaesthesia and Pain Management, University of Leicester at Leicester Royal Infirmary

Karen H. Simpson FRCA, Consultant Anaesthetist, St James's University Hospital, Leeds

Robert Sneyd MA MB BChir MD FRCA, Professor of Anaesthesia, Peninsula Medical School, Plymouth

Richard A. Struthers FRCA, Consultant Anaesthetist, Derriford Hospital, Plymouth

Trudy Towell MPhil, Nurse Consultant, Queen's Medical Centre, University Hospital, Nottingham

Andrew P. Vickers MB BS FRCA Consultant in Anaesthetics and Pain Management, Royal Lancaster Infirmary

Preface

Studies into patients' experiences of anaesthesia and surgery suggest that avoidance of post-operative nausea and vomiting (PONV) is a high priority for them but review of the literature on individual factors contributing to PONV is complicated by a lack of standardisation of the definitions of 'nausea' and 'vomiting' and frequently by the failure to control other factors that may contribute to this distressing and sometimes debilitating condition. Over ten years ago, in reflecting on the aetiology of PONV, Andrews posed the question: 'Why is the mechanism not known?', but at the time of writing – September 2003 – we remain almost equally ignorant of the precise physiological and pathophysiological mechanisms underlying its clinical manifestation although predisposing factors such as opiates and motion sensitivity, for example, are now better characterised.

Recent studies of the effects of anaesthetics on ligand-gated ion channels such as the 5-HT$_3$ receptor provide insights into the mechanisms of PONV but although 5-HT$_3$ receptor antagonists (e.g. ondansetron, granisetron, dolasetron) have demonstrable efficacy in PONV, 5-HT$_3$ receptors (but not necessarily 5-HT) may not have such a significant role in PONV as they do in the acute phase of chemotherapy-induced emesis. As Palazzo and Strunin (1984) pointed out almost 20 years ago in a landmark review, a cardinal characteristic of PONV is its multi-factorial nature and hence multiple emetic inputs and these may be activated to differing degrees depending on the surgical/anaesthetic/medication regimen. It is precisely for this reason that there has been much recent interest in the development and use of what have come to be described as 'universal' or 'broad-spectrum' anti-emetics such as the neurokinin-1 receptor antagonists. In Chapter 1 of this second edition text, Andrews provides an elegant description of the clinical studies of such agents against the background of the larger body of preclinical information that has accumulated and the insights they offer into the mechanism(s) of PONV.

Having reviewed the physiological mechanisms of PONV, Chapter 2 is concerned with the epidemiology of the condition, which Struthers and Sneyd conveniently discuss under the broad but entirely appropriate headings of 'patient', 'surgical' and 'anaesthetic' factors. Patient factors, as the authors outline, include age and sex, the phase of menstrual cycle, a previous history of PONV, motion sickness, smoking and obesity. Surgical factors, for example, are identified as including the nature of operation, children versus adults and the length of time during which surgery takes place. Anaesthetic factors will include the anaesthetist, the premedication and anaesthetic agents selected, neuromuscular blocking and reversal agents, peri-operative opioids, anaesthetic techniques, spinal anaesthesia, regional techniques, oxygenation, peri-operative hydration, post-operative pain and post-operative fluids. Not all these factors are, of course, likely to prove of equal importance. Indeed, with this in mind various approaches have been taken to predicting PONV, and most recently Apfel, for example, has demonstrated that a simple four-component scheme is as accurate as more elaborate equations. No system will, however, and as the authors point out, have a better than 70% chance of predicting PONV and they are clear that coupling of risk factors may well explain the apparent lack of additional predictive power of those scoring systems which employ multiple variables.

Having reviewed the physiological mechanisms and predicters of risk of PONV in Part One of the volume we have dedicated Part Two to the study of the evidentiary basis for pharmacological and non-pharmacological intervention in the prevention and management of the condition. In the first chapter of this part, Simpson reviews the role of alternative and complementary therapies in prophylaxis and management with particular emphasis on the evidence for, and role of, acupuncture techniques. In defence of the traditional methodological approaches employed in evaluating the efficacy and effectiveness of acupuncture, the author is keen to point out that clinical trials of acupuncture have required a quite different set of methodological assumptions than those that form the conceptual and methodological basis of classical drug trials. She importantly reminds the reader that the greatest number of published studies have been conducted in adult females, with questions therefore remaining over whether or not this technique is equally effective in adult males and, indeed, children (although her qualified conclusion based on the relatively smaller numbers of studies in these populations is that it is). She goes on to provide an impressive listing of the various studies that, taken together as a whole, certainly suggest that acupuncture can in given clinical circumstances represent an effective treatment for PONV, particularly as a useful alternative or adjunct to multi-modal anti-emetic therapy.

In the chapter that follows, Harmer provides a particularly thorough overview of the pharmacological prevention and control of PONV. Whereas patient and extraneous factors may influence the input into the process, most therapy is, as the author points out, aimed at the various receptor sites involved in the process and thus the major categories of drugs may be divided into anti-dopaminergic, anti-cholinergic, anti-histaminic, anti-serotonergic and anti-neurokininergic classes. The anti-dopaminergic drugs include, of course, metoclopramide, alizapride, droperidol, haloperidol and the phenothiazines, drugs that have variable efficacy in the management of PONV with some showing more preventative activity and others better effects as direct treatments but all having potentially problematic extra-pyramidal side-effects. Based on the receptor arguments, anti-cholinergic drugs should theoretically have a role to play but only hyoscine, as Harmer points out, has been shown to have any effect on nausea and vomiting and then only when the predisposing factor is vestibular in origin, while anti-histaminic drugs have been shown to be effective in travel sickness, only cyclizine has been shown to be effective in the treatment of PONV. Of the remaining classes that the author discusses, anti-serotonergic drugs have been shown to be highly effective in the prevention and treatment of nausea and vomiting associated with chemotherapy and although their efficacy in PONV is not as impressive they may nevertheless be particularly useful in prevention or treatment of the condition in the patient refractory to other classes of drugs. The most recent class of drug to have excited interest in the prevention and management of PONV is the neurokinin receptor antagonist, which has been shown by animal studies to prevent the vomiting process and where a role has recently been established in the management of chemotherapy-induced emesis in man. Research in relation to the place of NK-1 receptor antagonists in the prevention and management of PONV is ongoing and its results are awaited with much interest.

It is clear from Harmer's review that no one agent has proved consistently effective in preventing and managing PONV and treatment failure may occur in an individual patient or in a particular patient group. In such a scenario, combination therapy aimed at inhibition of multiple receptor pathways may well represent the most effective basis of treatment and it to the efficacy of this approach to therapy that Awad and Rowbotham turn in Chapter 5. The authors pose the question: 'What if anti-emetic therapy fails?', and in answer provide a useful list of suggestions for clinical practice. Consider, they argue, whether the patient has actually received the medication, that the dose was appropriate and that the absorption of the drug was likely. Persistent PONV, as they point out, may be associated with significant pathology and this needs to be identified and treated, with causes including hypotension, hypoxaemia, the use of antibiotics or other drugs, the inappropriate or insufficient use of opioids, pain, optimistic fluid intake and postoperative mobility, intestinal stasis and a range of psychological factors. Complicating the advice that can be given within the context of the authors' question is the paucity of well-designed trials in patients not responding to anti-emetic therapy, which are very difficult to perform. The authors are nevertheless clear that pathophysiological reasoning can be applied in clinical decision making where evidence does not exist to inform it and that when one anti-emetic fails it makes perfect sense to employ an additional drug that has a different mechanism of action compared with the first. Indeed, in much the same way as balanced analgesia provides improved pain relief, it is likely that the same approach could improve anti-emesis. Evidence, as Awad and Rowbotham describe, is emerging from the literature to support the contention that various combinations of anti-emetics can act synergistically, and these authors provide one of the most useful reviews of the pharmacological basis and clinical use of the various combination treatment regimens available to the anaesthetic team to have been published in recent years.

The complexity of anti-emetic drug administration and the increasing use of combination approaches to therapy described within Chapters 4 and 5 highlight the need to consider the pharmaceutical considerations that arise in the preparation and administration of anti-emetic agents. It is precisely to these that Howard turns in Chapter 6 of the volume which concludes Part Two of the text. The preparation of injectable anti-emetics, as Howard reminds us, is associated with several potential problems, the most immediate of which is the potential for particulate and microbial contamination. Although all injectables have particulate contamination, those given intravenously have the potential to cause organ damage through capillary blockage in the lungs, liver and kidneys. Filters, as the author points out, can prevent particulate matter reaching the systemic circulation and the choice of filter needle or terminal in-line filter will depend on the type of line being used or other agents that are being administered. As part of these considerations it is particularly important that preparation occurs under strict aseptic conditions and that injections should be prepared immediately before use, remembering that infusions have the greatest potential bacterial growth period and should therefore be made in an aseptic suite or bought as a ready to use product. Propofol, for example, is an ideal bacterial growth medium and for this reason should not have any other agents added to it. In terms of route of administration, Howard believes intramuscular injection to be far from ideal given the slow and erratic absorption profile of agents given by this route and also because of its association with tissue damage and pain, especially if the injection volume is greater than 2 mL. Where intravenous bolus administration is indicated, this should invariably be given according to the manufacturer's instructions and where anti-emetics need to be mixed with other agents, for example to preclude repeated intramuscular injections or in PCA syringes, mixing should never occur unless data exist on compatibility. For colleagues bewildered by the range of considerations listed, Howard would point out that resources exist within the hospital pharmacy department both for checking drug compatibility and when considering applying information to situations involving different concentrations of agents.

We have dedicated Part Three of the volume to a consideration of the clinical governance of PONV services and therefore to issues of quality assurance and quality improvement in routine clinical practice and within the context of an increasingly multi-disciplinary clinical team. Vickers, in addressing these issues, is clear that the optimal management of PONV must be considered a process that involves the identification of high-risk patients, the minimization of triggering factors, the appropriate prescription of anti-emetics both prophylactically and as treatment, the identification of established PONV and prompt institution of treatment, the audit of these objectives, the use of education programmes and guidelines to achieve these objectives, and the support of research to help to refine our understanding of the use and shortcomings of current medications and advance the development of new agents. In illustration of his arguments this author reviews the results of a 1999 survey of UK-wide practices for the management of PONV, comparing and contrasting the results gained with those derived from a later study in 2002 aimed at establishing whether or not any changes in practices had occurred over time. The results provide interesting lessons for the reader and it is worth reviewing some of the more salient findings here. In 1999, nearly three-quarters of respondents indicated that they had conducted some form of audit of PONV in their hospital, but less than half had done so in 2001. Fifty-one per cent felt they had an idea of the incidence of PONV in their hospital in

1999 but only about one-third agreed in 2002. Teaching was provided by 62% of respondents for new anaesthetists and by 65% for nurses but new non-anaesthetist doctors fared less well, with 39% of respondents educating them on the management of PONV in the 1999 survey. In 2002 these figures were 70%, 93% and 64% respectively. The use of guidelines, Vickers notes, was found to be very variable, ranging from 84% for treating PONV in adult in-patients (53% in 1999) but only 48% for treating children (31% in 1999). PONV was still considered to be a problem for in-patients even in these hospitals, where only 24% felt it was well managed (30% in 1999) although the figures for day cases were more positive at 62% (35% in 1999). Taken together, the results of the surveys showed that there is a wide variation in practices for the prevention and management of PONV in the UK, and many enthusiasts felt that PONV remains a problem in their hospital.

Although these results derive from only two surveys, the limitations of both of which were acknowledged by their authors, they nevertheless indicate that much remains to be done if real improvements in the quality of PONV services are to be achieved and sustained. In Chapter 8, which completes Part Three of the volume, Hobbs and colleagues are clear that, as with post-operative pain, poor organisation is the foundation for poor outcomes from the management of PONV. These authors argue that the introduction of a comprehensive strategy to re-organise PONV management can improve outcomes but that the success of a new clinical strategy will depend on effective contributions from all staff making clinical decisions and delivering patient care throughout the surgical or 'PONV' pathway. The strategy, they contend, should be able to get relevant research evidence, expert opinion and the practical experience of other leading teams into clinical practice, but they do not underestimate the task at hand and acknowledge that achieving this degree of organisational change and demonstrating and maintaining improvements in PONV outcomes will prove to be a continuing challenge. Interestingly, the authors highlight the nursing interventions in assessment, prevention and treatment of PONV, and support the pivotal role of the multi-disciplinary clinical team in implementing a comprehensive PONV management strategy. One such strategy and its outcomes are described, including suggestions for clinical practice guidelines and their discussion of the role of audit in implementing and maintaining organisational change and practice is of particular importance.

Part Four, the concluding part of the volume, has been dedicated to a discussion of future research strategies for the prevention and treatment of PONV. In Chapter 9, the final chapter, Hopkins addresses the 'gaps' in what might be termed the 'evidence landscape' for the understanding of PONV. His argument that an incidence of PONV of up to 70% in some surgical groups should dictate that research into the prevention and treatment of PONV has a high priority is of course compelling, and he echoes Andrews in Chapter 1 in lamenting the lack of efficacy of current therapies as a product of our current lack of understanding of the detailed neurophysiology of emetic reflexes.

Despite the deficiencies of animal models as paradigms of human emesis, Hopkins argues that basic research should nevertheless be pursued through which important knowledge could be obtained; for example, about the pathways and neurotransmitters involved in opioid-induced vomiting, about whether anaesthetics induce vomiting through actions at specific receptors or through non-specific actions, and whether there is a final common pathway for all emetic stimuli. Clinical research, the author contends, is clearly also warranted and further research has the potential to identify optimal regimens of the currently available therapies. As he points out, we are still unclear about the best dose (balancing wanted and unwanted effects) and timing of administration of many of the drugs currently available for clinical use and a more detailed analysis of the efficacy of individual drugs in relation to presumed triggers of PONV in the form of randomised controlled comparisons of available drugs would enable better targeting of treatment. There is, of course, much logic to the use of combinations of anti-emetics acting at different receptors as indeed has been discussed earlier in the text, and we join with Hopkins in calling for further randomised controlled trials of different combinations in studies necessarily employing large patient samples in a multi-centre approach. The outcome of such trials would be, as he points out, identification of optimal treatment strategies and these should be subjected to health economic evaluation and audit of efficacy.

In this second edition text we have aimed both to update previously published chapters and to include new contributions while maintaining the volume as concise as possible but as comprehensive as necessary. Anaesthetists, clinical nurse specialists in anaesthetics and hospital pharmacists are likely to find the volume of central significance to continuing professional development and we advance it specifically as an excellent tool for this purpose. We anticipate that the book will function additionally as a reference tool for colleagues working in surgery, theatre recovery and intensive care, and for academics and health services researchers working across all of these disciplines as well as medical and nursing students in their clinical years.

In conclusion, we thank Roche Products Ltd and GlaxoSmithKline UK Ltd for the grants of unrestricted educational sponsorship which helped fund a national symposium organised with The Royal College of Anaesthetists and the Association of Anaesthetists of Great Britain and Ireland at The Royal College of Physicians of London and which have additionally enabled us to ensure a particularly wide-ranging dissemination of this clinical text across the UK as a major contribution to the development of effective clinical practice.

Leo Strunin MD FRCA FRCPC
David Rowbotham MD MRCP FRCA
Andrew Miles MSc MPhil PhD

PART 1

Mechanisms, epidemiology and risk

Approaching an understanding of the mechanism of post-operative nausea and vomiting

Paul L.R. Andrews

Introduction

As anaesthesia and surgery have become progressively safer procedures, attention has focused on other consequences which may reduce quality of life and delay recovery (e.g. disturbed gut function (Herbert *et al.* 1999)), resulting in a longer hospital stay.

The treatment of post-operative nausea and vomiting (PONV) is still a major challenge for patient management, although advances have been and continue to be made in understanding its underlying mechanisms. This chapter will focus on some aspects of PONV to illustrate not only areas in which progress is being made but also areas of neglect and ignorance.

Why PONV?

The emetic system is remarkable in that it can respond to diverse chemical stimuli, many of which are very unlikely to have been present in the environment during the course of evolution at least until recently. In the wild, nausea and vomiting subserved defensive functions to protect the body against toxins ingested accidentally with the food (Andrews 1993). A fundamental question to understanding PONV is to identify how particular elements of the operative environment can (unfortunately) trigger this defensive reflex.

The unpleasant sensation of nausea stops further ingestion of contaminated food (cf. 'warning' function of pain) and, probably of greater importance, leads to the formation of a learned or conditioned aversion. This links the taste, smell or sight of the food to a memory of the sensation of nausea which it induced on the previous occasion. Such conditioned aversions may only require a single exposure for induction and can last for many years, if not a lifetime. Many of the readers of this chapter will be able to identify foods which made them ill, particularly as a child, and which they will still not eat.

Aversive responses may also be induced by stimuli in the clinical environment, with the best characterised example being the response to anticancer chemotherapy drugs, such as cisplatin. Patients who experience nausea and vomiting as a side-effect during the first or subsequent cycles of treatment may develop anticipatory nausea and vomiting with the prevalence being about 25% (Morrow *et al.* 1998). This may take the form of the induction of nausea or even vomiting by the receipt of a hospital appointment card, the sight of the hospital, the smell of the hospital or even the sight of the staff involved in administration of the chemotherapy in a non-clinical setting (e.g. supermarket). While post-operative nausea is not usually as severe or protracted as anti-cancer chemotherapy-induced nausea and vomiting, it has the same potential for inducing aversive and anticipatory responses. Even if an aversion is not induced, it is likely that each time the emetic system is activated the organism 'learns' from the experience. These experiences will contribute to the overall 'emetic history' of the individual, which in turn may influence the probability of whether the individual will have nausea or vomiting in a particular clinical setting (e.g. chemotherapy, PONV).

The function of vomiting is to forcibly expel material in bulk from the upper gastrointestinal tract. The vomiting response to ingested toxins is self-limiting, provided that it has been detected before absorption, in that the toxin responsible for initiating the response is removed by the act which it triggers (i.e. vomiting). In contrast, when the emetic stimulus is in the blood stream as is the case in many clinical situations (e.g. anti-cancer chemotherapy) vomiting will not remove it from the body and the response will be protracted with the duration depending upon metabolism and excretion (Andrews & Davis 1995).

To summarise, the reason why PONV occurs is that some feature(s) of the operative environment is able to activate one or more of the inputs to the emetic system, which itself evolved to eject toxins via the mouth and by the genesis of nausea and aversions to learn from the experience. The clinical importance of learning and plasticity in the emetic system (Andrews *et al.* 1990b) have been relatively neglected. Consideration should be given to taking a complete 'emetic history' as each time the system is activated it will influence the subsequent response even if the stimulus is different.

Physiology of nausea and vomiting

Pathways for activation and integration of the emetic reflex

The majority of our knowledge of the pathways by which vomiting can be induced comes from studies of animal models (e.g. dog, cat, ferret, house musk shrew, but not rats, mice and rabbits, which do not vomit) and perhaps with the exception of the psychological and cerebral influences the same pathways operate as in humans.

The pathways have been studied using retching and vomiting as endpoints, as nausea is difficult to study in animals (see below) although it can be induced by activation of the same pathways that can induce vomiting. However, while retching and vomiting are generated by brainstem mechanisms, the genesis of nausea requires the presence of higher brain regions (Figure 1.1).

The major pathways by which the emetic reflex can be induced have been identified (see Andrews 1993 and Andrews & Davis 1995 for reviews):

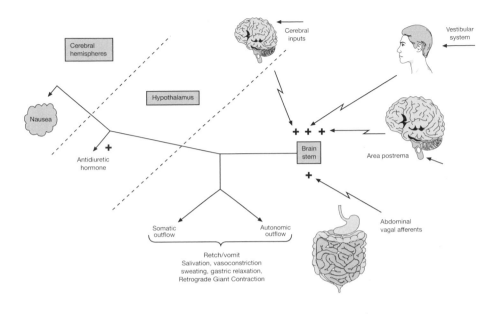

Figure 1.1 Diagrammatic representation of pathways for the induction of nausea and vomiting.

- abdominal vagal afferents
- area postrema
- vestibular system.

Abdominal vagal afferents

Most axons in the abdominal vagi are afferent (approx. 80–90%) conveying information from the gut to the brainstem (primarily the nucleus tractus solitarius) about the degree of distension and contractile activity of the muscle (mechanoreceptors) (Grundy & Scratcherd 1989) and features of the luminal environment, such as osmolarity, pH and the shearing of contents against the mucosa (chemoreceptors). These afferents play a role in the daily regulation of the gastrointestinal motor and secretory responses to food. Both types of afferent can induce emesis when appropriately triggered with the signal having intensity (high frequency) and temporal (prolonged activation) domains to prevent 'accidental' triggering of the emetic reflex. Using electrical stimulation which activates the axons synchronously, retching can be induced in the anaesthetised animal in less than 20 seconds (Andrews *et al.* 1990b).

A considerable body of experimental evidence shows that the activation of the vagal afferent signalling information from the mucosa is indirect via the release of neuroactive agents such as 5-hydroxytryptamine (5-HT) and cholecystokinin (CCK) from enteroendocrine cells (Grundy & Scratcherd 1989; Andrews & Davis 1995; Hillsey & Grundy 1998). It is proposed that systemic cytotoxic drugs (e.g. cisplatin) and radiation used in the treatment of cancer induce the exocytotic release of 5-HT from the enterochromaffin (EC) cells via the generation of free radicals and the influx of calcium ions. The 5-HT acts on $5-HT_3$ receptors (a ligand-gated ion channel) located on vagal afferents terminating in close proximity to discharge the afferent and provide an emetic signal to the brainstem (Andrews & Davis 1995). The major site of action of the $5-HT_3$ receptor antagonists (e.g. granisetron, ondansetron) used in the treatment of chemotherapy-induced emesis is proposed to be on the peripheral vagal afferent terminals to block the effects of 5-HT (Andrews & Davis 1995). The role of other neuroactive agents in the induction of emesis by activation of vagal afferents has not been investigated but their involvement could account for the less than complete blockade of acute nausea and vomiting by $5-HT_3$ receptor antagonists in some chemo- and radiotherapy patients.

Appropriate activation of the abdominal vagal afferents can readily induce retching and vomiting, while similar stimulation of the greater splanchnic nerve does not (Andrews *et al.* 1990b). The role of the splanchnic afferents in the genesis of nausea is unclear but these afferents convey noxious sensations and nausea is associated with pain (Desbiens *et al.* 1997). A study in humans has shown that sympathetic activation heightens the perception of experimental induced distension (Iovino *et al.* 1995). Sympathetic activation is associated with nausea and hence sympathetically mediated heightened perception could contribute to the epigastric awareness reported in nausea.

Experimental studies of the emetic reflex have provided evidence of plasticity (Andrews *et al.* 1990b). These observations come from experiments in which the acute section of the abdominal vagi but not the greater splanchnic nerves abolishes the emetic response to a particular challenge (e.g. radiation) indicating a critical role for the vagi. However, when animals are tested several weeks later with the same emetic stimulus, a response is present. There is some indication that the splanchnic afferents may mediate the response but in other studies section of the splanchnic nerves failed to abolish the response leading to the suggestion that it was mediated by the release of a substance from the gut, entering the circulation to act on the area postrema (see below) (Andrews *et al.* 1992; Makale & King 1993).

Area postrema

The area postrema is a circumventricular organ located at the caudal extremity of the floor of the fourth ventricle in the region of the obex (Leslie & Reynolds 1991). The blood brain barrier is permeable in this region making it structurally adapted for the detection of circulating substances, including peptides, from the gut. Ablation studies (including in humans) (Lindstrom & Brizzee 1962) have implicated the area postrema in emesis and have led to it being termed the 'chemoreceptor trigger zone' (CTZ) for emesis. This terminology has led to the erroneous assumption that any substance in the circulation which causes emesis must do so via the area postrema (Leslie & Reynolds 1992). The area postrema has been implicated by ablation studies in the emesis induced by opiate and dopamine receptor agonists but recent studies have suggested that the site of action may not be the area postrema but receptors on dendrites of the subjacent nucleus tractus solitarius (NTS), which project into the area postrema. The area postrema may thus be envisaged as providing a window to the NTS and lesions of the area postrema would inevitably cause collateral damage to the NTS, the major site of projection of vagal afferents. The role of the area postrema thus needs to be reassessed.

Vestibular system

The vestibular labyrinths provide the pathway for the induction of motion sickness (Koch 1993) with the disparity between the input from the visual and vestibular systems providing a potent signal. However, although blind people may become motion sick, those with severe bilateral labyrinthine damage do not. The function and evolutionary relevance (if any) of motion sickness is unclear but the vestibular input into the brainstem appears to be of importance in modifying the sensitivity of the emetic reflex. For example, head position in healthy volunteers has been shown to influence the emetic response to apomorphine acting via the brainstem (Isaacs 1957).

Other pathways

The emetic reflex can be activated from a number of other sites but they have been less well studied in contrast to the above inputs. Both nausea and vomiting can be induced by electrical stimulation of the discrete regions of the cerebral hemispheres (Sem-Jacobsen 1968). The natural stimulus for activation is not known but it appears likely that this is the route by which psychogenic stimuli induce nausea and vomiting. It is not known if any drugs act here to induce nausea and vomiting. A probable role for these cerebral outputs is to modulate the sensitivity of the brainstem mechanisms.

Nausea and vomiting can be induced by activation of a population of cardiac ventricular vagal afferents, auricular vagal afferents and pharyngeal afferents (Andrews & Davis 1995). They may also be induced by visual, olfactory and gustatory inputs but it is unclear whether this is a learned response.

Nausea

The subjective nature of the sensation of nausea has made it difficult to study the mechanisms involved in its genesis, particularly in animals. There are no objective measures of nausea in humans which do not rely on self-report by the patient. Production of the sensation obviously requires activation of neural pathways, which eventually project to areas of the cerebral hemispheres dealing with conscious sensations. The question remains as to how these pathways are activated and whether the visceral awareness (particularly abdominal) which accompanies nausea is direct or referred.

Studies using motion as the stimulus suggest that nausea is induced by lower levels of activation of the inputs to the emetic pathway(s) than are required to induce vomiting (Koch 1993). This model would be consistent with the 'warning' function of nausea. Attempts to understand the mechanisms underlying nausea and to identify objective markers have focused on the endocrine, gastric and autonomic nervous system-mediated changes which accompany it.

Endocrine changes

These can be divided into those which occur as a component of the response to a stressful stimulus and those which appear specific to nausea. In the latter category plasma vasopressin (ADH, AVP) is the best example (Nussey *et al.* 1988; Koch 1995, 1997). Massive (>50× maximal anti-diuretic levels in some studies) increases in vasopressin, but not oxytocin, have been reported in close temporal association with the onset and continued presence of nausea induced by illusory self-motion, oral ipecac, systemic apomorphine, cholecystokinin and anti-cancer chemotherapy drugs (e.g. cisplatin). Unfortunately, there do not appear to be any studies in patients with PONV. Such studies would be of interest but care would be needed to control for the degree of hydration. One function of the ADH would be to promote fluid conservation in anticipation of the expected fluid loss which will occur if vomiting and diarrhoea ensue but the magnitude of the rise suggests that it may have other functions. When present in high concentrations in the plasma, vasopressin, as its name implies, can have vasoconstrictor effects. Such effects could reduce GI tract blood flow and also contribute to cutaneous vasoconstriction, resulting in the characteristic pallor of nauseated individuals. The effects of high concentrations of ADH on the gut are not well described but, by analogy with its constrictor effect on vascular smooth muscle, some elevation in tone is likely. This could account for the diffuse abdominal sensations which accompany nausea if the motor changes activated abdominal visceral afferents. High levels of circulating vasopressin could also have an effect on the area postrema (see above) to activate pathways projecting from the nucleus tractus solitarius to more rostral parts of the brain, either generating the sensation of nausea or acting in concert with another input.

Gastric motor changes

The most consistent alteration in gastric physiology associated with the presence of nausea is an increase in the gastric electrical slow wave frequency from ~3 c.p.m. to 4–9 c.p.m. (Koch 1995; 1997). This has been extensively studied in subjects exposed to illusory self-motion (vection) where the frequency increased prior to the onset of reported nausea. Similar frequency increases have also been observed during the first trimester of pregnancy and in patients with diabetic or idiopathic gastroparesis, functional dyspepsia, peptic ulcer disease and those undergoing abdominal surgery. It is unclear whether the dysrhythmias contribute to the genesis of the sensation of nausea (via activation of afferents) or whether they are secondary to the complex endocrine (e.g. adrenaline, β endorphin, ADH) or autonomic changes which accompany nausea and stressful events. One study of tachygastrias in patients following major abdominal surgery failed to show a difference between the patients with and without PONV (Clevers *et al.* 1992). This suggests that the tachygastrias are induced by features of the operative environment but do not cause PONV. The presence of tachygastrias may be a predisposing or priming factor for the induction of PONV, with additional factors required for its expression.

Autonomic nervous system-mediated changes

Many of the signs which accompany nausea are mediated by the autonomic nervous system (Andrews 1999a) and are indicative of a generalised autonomic arousal as might be expected due to the generally stressful nature of the experience. These include overt salivation frequently accompanied by repetitive swallowing (and aerophagy?), tachycardia, an increase in heart inter-beat interval variability, pupil dilatation, cutaneous vasoconstriction and sweating, giving rise to the pallor and the cold clammy feel of the skin. However, there is no evidence that any of the above give rise to the sensation of nausea, although they may contribute to the general discomfort of the patient.

In conclusion, the mechanisms underlying the genesis of nausea are relatively poorly understood, although recent imaging studies have demonstrated activation of the inferior frontal gyrus in subjects nauseated by vestibular stimulation or oral syrup of ipecac (Miller *et al.* 1996). Further imaging studies particularly in nauseated patients are required to identify if one particular region of the cerebral hemispheres is implicated.

Retching and vomiting

In contrast to nausea the mechanisms generating retching and vomiting and temporally related events are relatively well understood (Figure 1.2).

Shortly before the onset of retching preparatory changes have taken place in the gastrointestinal tract (Lang 1990; Lang *et al.* 1993). Relaxation of the proximal stomach occurs mediated by suppression of activity in vagal efferents supplying intrinsic cholinergic neurones and an increase in activity in the vagal efferents supplying the non-cholinergic, non-adrenergic intrinsic inhibitory neurons. The latter use vasoactive intestinal polypeptide and nitric oxide as their neurotransmitter. The relaxation is proposed to have three functions: to reduce emptying of potentially contaminated gastric contents into the duodenum; to place the proximal stomach in an optimum mechanical position for compression by the abdominal muscles and diaphragm during vomiting; and to accommodate refluxed intestinal contents.

Immediately before the initiation of retching a contraction is initiated in the mid-small intestine which sweeps retrogradely towards the stomach. This 'retrograde giant

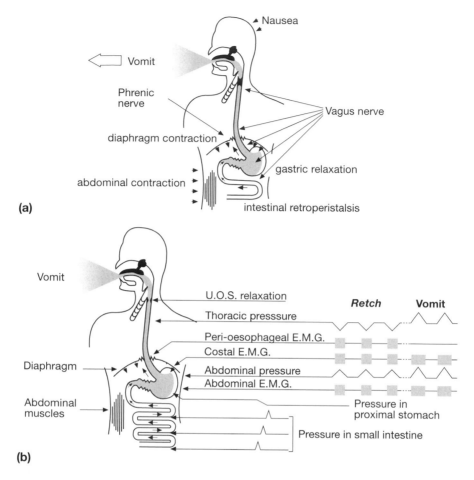

Figure 1.2 Major motor pathways (a) and motor components of vomiting (b).

contraction' (RGC) is under vagal cholinergic control and can be blocked by atropine. The primary function of the RGC is to return intestinal contents, which may be contaminated, to the stomach from where they can be expelled by vomiting. It has also been proposed that pancreatic juice will enter the stomach by the RGC and may serve to buffer the acidic gastric contents prior to vomiting. The RGC probably accounts for the frequent presence of bile in the stomach. During surgery bile may also enter the stomach if gastroduodenal motility is disrupted. The irritant nature of bile may provide a further emetic drive by stimulation of the mucosal afferents.

Retching begins when the RGC reaches the stomach, marking the end of the prodromal or pre-ejection phase and the beginning of the ejection phase. However, the RGC is not essential for its initiation, as retching will occur even if the RGC is blocked either by atropine or abdominal vagotomy.

Retching is frequently referred to as 'unproductive vomiting' or 'attempts to vomit' and while both expressions are true, retching and vomiting are distinct but related processes (Koga & Fukuda 1990; Grelot & Miller 1996). During retching the anterior abdominal muscles (e.g. oblique, rectus and transverse abdominis muscles) and all parts of the diaphragm contract synchronously and rhythmically, whereas during vomiting there is more intense and prolonged activation of all the muscles except the perioesophageal (crural) diaphragm, which does not contract. In addition, during vomiting a retrograde contraction occurs in the striated muscle portion of the oesophagus and the upper oesophageal sphincter is widely opened by intense activation of the geniohyoid muscle (Minami *et al.* 1995; Grelot & Miller 1996). Thus the major expulsive force for vomiting is generated by compression of the stomach by contraction of the abdominal muscles and the descending diaphragm. During retching and vomiting a characteristic posture is usually adopted presumably to optimise the compression of the stomach and perhaps prevent strain of some muscle groups.

The function of retching is unclear and, as vomiting can occur without prior retching, it is clearly not an essential prerequisite. It has been proposed that retching helps overcome the anti-reflux barrier in the region of the lower oesophageal sphincter and to impart momentum to the gastric contents for expulsion. The factors regulating the number of retches preceding a vomit are unclear, although animal studies have shown that the number of retches is influenced by gastric volume, with low volumes increasing the number of retches preceding a vomit (Andrews *et al.* 1990a). What determines the transition from retching to a vomit is unclear, although blood gas levels have been implicated (Fukuda & Koga 1993).

The somatic and autonomic nervous system-mediated events are co-ordinated in the brainstem. The term 'vomiting centre' is a convenient shorthand term for the co-ordinating system but in reality the motor pattern is probably generated by a network of nuclei with perhaps the nucleus tractus solitarius and the central respiratory pattern generator playing predominant roles (Grelot & Miller 1996; Koga *et al.* 1998).

Emetic stimuli in the operative environment

The operative environment is complex, containing numerous potentially emetic stimuli. It is the interaction of these stimuli both with each other and with the individual patient which will determine whether a patient will experience PONV. Within this complex environment it is probable that some factors will have a greater effect than others and their removal would be expected to have a significant effect on the incidence of PONV. Epidemiological studies have played an increasingly important role in identifying several risk factors for the induction of PONV. As a result, they have provided important insights into some of the underlying mechanisms (see, for example, Palazzo & Strunin 1984; Watcha & White 1992; Apfel *et al.* 1999, 2001, 2002a, b). The major risk factors are: female gender; history of motion sickness or PONV; non-smoking; use of post-operative opioids; inhalational anaesthesia. The last factor has been shown to be the main one involved in emesis in the early (0–2 hours) as opposed to the later (2–24 hours) period after surgery and anaesthesia (Apfel *et al.* 2002a). This study is also important in identifying PONV as a heterogeneous phenomenon and hence it may be unrealistic to expect that a single mechanism is involved.

In this chapter we will attempt to explain how some features of the operative environment may trigger this primitive protective reflex. It is not possible to review all the factors but they have been reviewed more extensively elsewhere (Palazzo & Strunin 1984; Andrews 1992, 1999b; Watcha & White 1992).

Pre-operative factors

The previous emetic history of the patient will influence the response to subsequent emetic stimuli, as each time the emetic system is activated the patient will 'learn' from the experience. There is also a growing recognition that a patient's expectation of whether or not they will have emesis can influence the impact of anti-emetics (Eden & Zuk 1995). The use of such 'verbal-placebos' requires further investigation, particularly to identify the intrinsic mechanisms which are accessed by such interventions. Individual differences in emetic sensitivity, which suggest that there is likely to be a genotype which predisposes to an emetic phenotype, have probably been underestimated (Xu *et al.* 1993). There is some evidence for racial differences in emetic sensitivity and gender differences in emetic sensitivity are well described in humans, with females being more sensitive – although in some other species (e.g. the house musk shrew) the male is more sensitive to some emetic stimuli (Matsuki *et al.* 1997). In addition, 'environmental' factors, such as high alcohol intake, are protective against anti-cancer chemotherapy-induced emesis (D'Acquisto *et al.* 1986). Tobacco smoking is a particularly interesting risk factor for PONV because it is protective, in contrast to other factors (Apfel *et al.* 1999; Chimbira and Sweeney 2000). Although there is some evidence that smoking during pregnancy may reduce pregnancy sickness (Gadsby *et al.* 1997) little is known about its impact upon other emetic challenges.

The mechanism by which smoking has this effect has not been elucidated but several mechanisms have been hypothesised: tobacco may contain an anti-emetic substance (Chimbira & Sweeney 2000); smoking may affect the dopaminergic system in the brain (Apfel *et al.* 1997); induction of cytochrome P450 enzymes in the liver or brain (Chimbira & Sweeney 2000). It is particularly puzzling that tobacco smoking should be protective, as nicotine is a potent emetic agent. Nausea and vomiting can be adverse events in nicotine-patch users, with the incidence being reduced by tapering the dose (Greenland *et al.* 1998). New smokers often report nausea. The neuronal nicotinic acetylcholine receptor is a ligand-gated ion channel belonging to the same family as the 5-HT$_3$ receptor. It is conceivable that although an 'acute' exposure to nicotine leads to activation of central emetic pathways more 'chronic' exposure leads to a desensitisation of the central emetic pathways. Such a mechanism would be supported if it is found that smoking is protective against a range of emetic stimuli acting at central and peripheral sites. In addition, it should be possible to mimic the effects of smoking by the use of nicotine patches in non-smokers. A study of the mechanism by which tobacco smoking protects against PONV (and perhaps other forms of emesis) may provide an insight into a novel approach to anti-emesis.

Two other patient-predictive factors have been identified in cancer patients undergoing chemotherapy; these may be relevant to PONV patients. Firstly, the magnitude of chemotherapy-induced nausea is inversely related to urinary cortisol secretion (Fredrikson et al. 1992). The reason why patients differ in their cortisol levels is unclear but is consistent with the finding that synthetic glucocorticoids have anti-emetic effects. Secondly, 'high' levels of night-time noradrenaline secretion were associated with an increased intensity of delayed nausea in cancer patients undergoing chemotherapy (Fredrikson et al. 1994).

One factor that is overlooked and to which consideration should be given is the reason for the surgery, as it is likely that the emetic reflex is sensitised in patients who have symptoms of nausea and vomiting caused by their illness (e.g. gastrointestinal, central nervous system or labyrinthine disease) or condition (e.g. early pregnancy).

Whereas all the above factors and others (e.g. glycaemic state, food, hydrational state) can predispose a patient to emesis during induction or post-operatively, they are not the cause of PONV, which must reside in stimuli to which the patient is exposed during surgery.

Peri- and intra-operative factors

The peri- and intra-operative environment provides a diverse range of mechanical and chemical emetic stimuli. Selected examples are discussed below.

Distension

Distension of the stomach and upper small intestine by a volatile anaesthetic could provide an emetic stimulus by activation of mechanoreceptors with afferents in the abdominal vagus. The most sensitive regions from which distension can induce nausea and eventually vomiting are those with little storage capacity such as the gastric antrum and the duodenum. During surgery, gas is more likely to accumulate because of the marked reduction in motility which occurs. It is not known if the ability of the stomach to relax is impaired during anaesthesia and surgery but belching to remove the gas may not be possible. It is unlikely that distension provides a major stimulus, however, it may act as a facilitatory factor as, until the gas is voided, the nucleus tractus solitarius (see above) will be receiving a continuous input from the vagal afferents and distension, particularly of the gastric fundus, promotes relaxation of the lower oesophageal sphincter via a vago-vagal reflex.

; of surgery (e.g. ENT) blood may enter the gastrointestinal tract and, frequently been commented that blood is emetic, the mechanism has not been investigated directly. The effect of blood is more likely to be due to its chemical nature rather than distension. However, the emetic effect of blood is puzzling as in some cultures (e.g. Masai of Tanzania) ingestion of fresh blood taken directly from the jugular veins of cattle or sheep forms part of the diet (Tannahill 1996). If blood is emetic, the most likely source of the stimulus is the cellular components which contain, or have the ability to synthesise, a number of neuroactive agents (e.g. dopamine, 5-HT, ATP, prostaglandins, cytokines). Release of such agents in close proximity to the mucosa could activate nerve ending in the mucosa directly or indirectly by stimulating the release of mediators from the enteroendocrine cells in the mucosa (see above). As with distension, prolonged mucosal irritation by accumulated blood will sensitise the central pathways to other stimuli adding to the overall 'emetic burden'.

Opioids

Opioids have a wide spectrum of pharmacological effects depending upon the particular agent and the dose. Dose-response studies of morphine in animals have shown that at 'low' doses it is emetic, whereas at 'high' doses its emetic effects reduce (Thompson *et al.* 1992) and it can be shown to have anti-emetic effects blocking the response to other emetic agents (e.g. copper sulphate, apomorphine, cyclophosphamide) (Rudd & Naylor 1995). The involvement of opioids in emesis is complex. The involvement of the various receptors (μ, δ, κ) has not been fully elucidated and studies have been complicated by species differences (Rudd & Naylor 1995). All three opioid receptors have been implicated in emesis by an action in the dorsal brainstem (area postrema and nucleus tractus solitarius), with perhaps μ_1 receptors having a major involvement. The anti-emetic effect of morphine and the emetic or pro-emetic effect of naloxone reported in several species, including humans, have been used as an indication that there is an 'anti-emetic centre' in the brainstem which can modulate the emetic reflex (Rudd & Naylor 1995). Identification of this region and its neurotransmitters would provide a novel target for anti-emetic drugs. Preclinical research has implicated μ_2 receptors in the anti-emetic effects of fentanyl. However, the site of action has still not been elucidated although the nucleus tractus solitarius appears a likely target (Rudd *et al.* 1999).

Clearly, morphine and related opioids could induce emesis by a direct central action if present when the patient emerges from general anaesthesia. However, opioids have other actions which could contribute to emesis by sensitising to other stimuli. For example, they can decrease gastric emptying, which may already be decreased by the use of muscarinic receptor antagonists, sensitise the vestibular system (opioids are more emetic in ambulatory patients), induce the release of ADH (see section on nausea, on page 7) and induce the release of 5-HT from the intestinal enterochromaffin cells (Racke & Schwoerer 1991). Each effect could induce nausea and vomiting if intense enough but, even if only activated to a low level, it would certainly contribute to the overall emetic burden to which the patient is exposed and perhaps sensitise to other emetic inputs.

It is perhaps timely to reassess the involvement of opioids in PONV as a number of agents other than morphine are in clinical use and understanding of opioid receptor pharmacology has improved as has clinical trials methodology. For example, a recent randomised, prospective and stratified study of patients undergoing strabismus or ENT surgery failed to demonstrate a statistically significant difference in PONV between patients who received low-dose opiates (fentanyl, sufentanil or alfentanil) or no opiate prior to induction of general anaesthesia (Kranke *et al.* 1998).

Anaesthetics

The recognition that neurotransmitter-gated ion channels (e.g. $GABA_A$, strychnine-sensitive glycine receptor, nicotinic acetylcholine receptor, ionotropic glutamate receptor) may be the molecular target for general anaesthetics suggests novel ways in which they may induce PONV (Peters & Lambert 1997) (Figure 1.3).

Several injectable (e.g. ketamine) as well as volatile anaesthetics (e.g. isoflurane, halothane) modulate the $5\text{-}HT_3$ receptor, although not all general anaesthetics have the same action. A positive allosteric modulation could be a significant factor in the genesis of PONV (Parker *et al.* 1996; Bentley & Barnes 1998). It is unlikely that such modulation of $5\text{-}HT_3$ receptors alone accounts for PONV, as blockade by selective antagonists would be expected to be more efficacious than is the case. However, the relevant site for the modulation is probably $5\text{-}HT_3$ receptors in the brainstem which are synaptically driven and, as the drugs used are competitive antagonists at the $5\text{-}HT_3$ receptor, higher doses may be required than are used to block the emetic response to anti-cancer chemotherapy agents, where the major site is peripheral (see above). It would be of interest to investigate whether the emesis induced by some anaesthetics is more amenable to treatment with $5\text{-}HT_3$ receptor antagonists than others.

There is continuing debate about whether propofol is intrinsically less emetic than other anaesthetic agents or whether it actually has anti-emetic properties. A study by Barann *et al.* (2000) of $5\text{-}HT_3$ receptors in a cell line showed that propofol in the micromolar range reduced currents induced by 5-HT activation of $5\text{-}HT_3$ receptors. The demonstration in the clinic that $5\text{-}HT_3$ receptor antagonists have some protective effects against PONV indicates that they are activated *in vivo*. If propofol inhibits the $5\text{-}HT_3$ receptor *in vivo* this could reduce nerve activity (or increase the threshold for activation) and hence the drive for emesis.

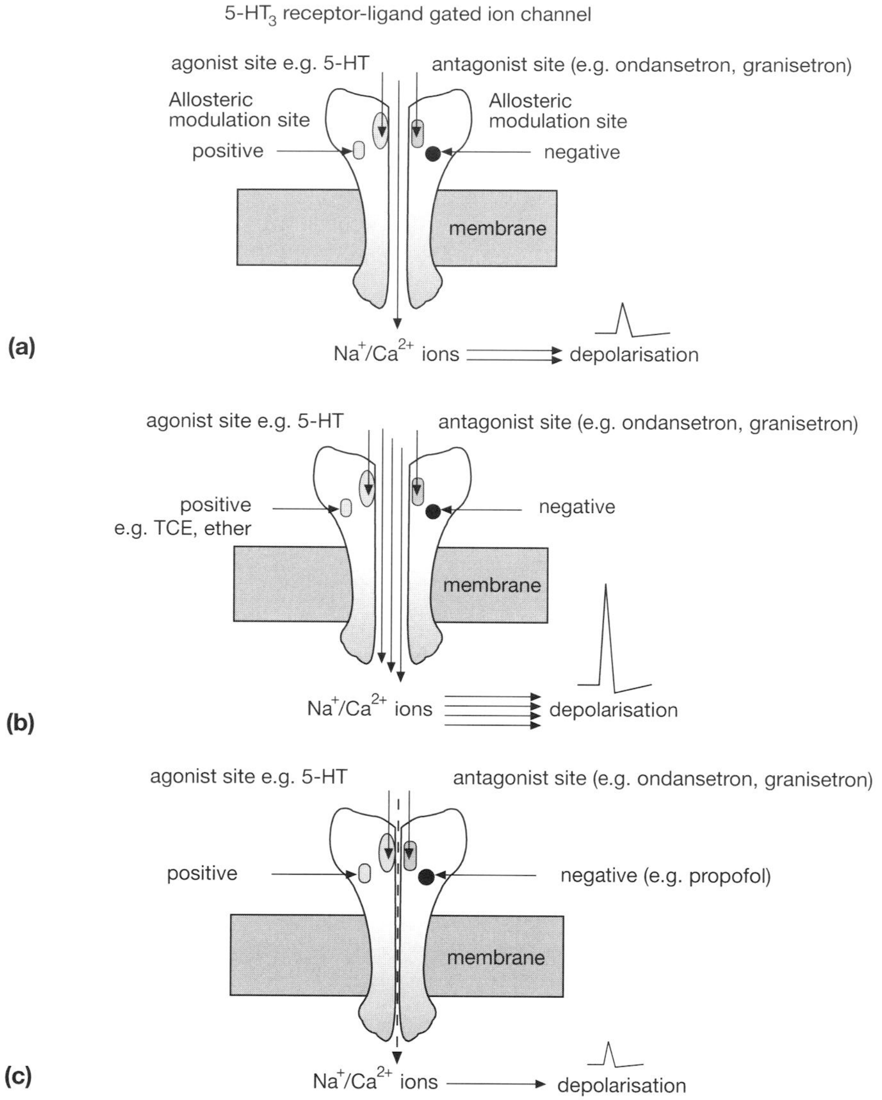

Figure 1.3 Diagram illustrating the possible involvement of the 5-Hydroxytryptamine$_3$ receptor (5-HT$_3$) in PONV.

Panel 'a' shows the basic structure of the 5-HT$_3$ receptor as a ligand-gated ion channel which when "open" allows the influx of Na$^+$ and Ca^{++} ions into the cell and efflux of K$^+$ (not shown) leading to depolarisation. The channel can be activated ("opened") when the agonist ligand (5-HT) binds to the agonist site. Binding of an antagonist such as ondansetron or granisetron to the antagonist site will block the action of the agonist. The receptor also has allosteric modulation sites which can either increase (positive site- e.g. TCE, ether, panel b) or decrease (negative site- e.g. propofol, panel c) activation of the receptor by the agonist (5-HT). It is proposed that 5-HT$_3$ receptors located on neurones in the emetic pathways (Figure 1.1) such as the nucleus tractus solitarius and abdominal vagal afferents have their activity modulated by certain anaesthetics leading to either an increase (positive modulation) or decrease (negative modulation) in the probability of emesis. This model could also account for the efficacy of 5-HT$_3$ receptor antagonists in PONV. See text for references.

Surgery

Surgery itself is perhaps the easiest stimulus to understand because it is evident that if the mechanical trauma of surgery activates one of the emetic pathways sufficiently, then emesis could result. However, this does not occur in normal clinical practice as the patient is anaesthetised and depending upon the type of surgery and national practice may have a neuromuscular blocking agent. These effects would be expected to be most marked during surgery but they probably persist into the post-operative period due to neuroactive agents released in response to local trauma (e.g. by damaged cells and axon reflexes). The unique nature of surgery in the experience of an animal should not be neglected as such trauma and manipulation of internal organs would only be experienced when an animal is being attacked!

Post-operative

It is in the post-operative period that nausea and vomiting occur. While the emetic stimuli are active during anaesthesia, the anaesthetic state suppresses but does not block the emetic pathway as intense activation of abdominal vagal afferents can induce retching even in deeply anaesthetised (i.e. absence of reflex withdrawal of a limb to a noxious stimulus) animals (Andrews & Davis 1995). From this it could be argued that the intra-operative emetic stimuli are not sufficiently intense. The suppression of the emetic reflex by general anaesthesia was used to reduce emesis in patients undergoing total body irradiation (Whitwam *et al.* 1978).

It is most likely that PONV results from an accumulation and persistence of the pre-, peri- and intra-operative factors but additional stimuli in the post-operative period may provide the final trigger. For example, on emergence from anaesthesia the patient will become aware of an altered state of consciousness and perception. While this may contribute to PONV, of arguably greater significance is motion.

During anaesthesia there is an absence of body, and particularly head, movement in comparison to sleep. Thus during surgery there will be an abnormally low input from the vestibular system which will become active as the patient is aroused, makes uncoordinated movements and is moved on a trolley, often in a semi-conscious state.

Pharmacology of emesis and anti-emetics (Figure 1.4)

Despite the large number of substances which are claimed to have anti-emetic properties, relatively little is known about the transmitters involved at key points in the emetic pathway. Care should be taken to distinguish between anti-emetics with direct effects blocking transmission at a critical point in the emetic pathway (e.g. NK_1 receptor antagonists, see below) and those which have an indirect action, such as alleviating gastric stasis (e.g. the $5\text{-}HT_4$ receptor agonist effect of metoclopramide) (Andrews 1994).

Because an agent has an anti-emetic effect in one condition, it does not necessarily follow that it will have an effect in another condition; some consideration must be given to the underlying cause and the pathway activated. This can be illustrated by the

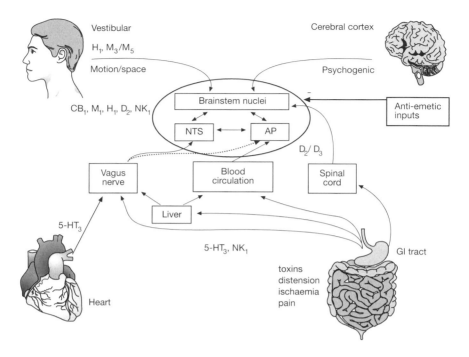

AP, area postrema; CB_1, Cannabinoid$_1$ receptor; D_2/D_3, dopamine$_{2/3}$ receptors; H_1, histamine$_1$ receptor; 5-HT$_3$, 5-Hydroxytryptamine$_3$ receptors; $M_{3/5}$, muscarinic$_{3/5}$ acetylcholine receptor; NK_1, neurokinin$_1$ (tachykinin) receptor; NTS, nucleus tractus solitarius.

Figure 1.4 Summary of aspects of the pharmacology of emesis and anti-emetics showing the major inputs by which emesis can be activated together with the major transmitter receptor systems involved. Redrawn and modified from Sanger and Andrews 2001

5-HT$_3$ receptor antagonists (Andrews 1994). These agents are very efficacious in the acute phase of anti-cancer chemotherapy-induced emesis because their primary site of action is to block the activation by 5-HT (released from the intestinal enterochromaffin cells by the chemotherapeutic agent) of the 5-HT$_3$ receptors located on the peripheral terminals of the vagal afferents. Any emetic stimulus acting via this pathway will have its effect reduced or blocked by a 5-HT$_3$ receptor antagonist. However, emetic stimuli acting via other mechanisms (e.g. motion, dopamine and opiate receptor agonists acting via the AP/NTS) will not be affected. 5-HT$_3$ receptors are present in the NTS but there is little preclinical evidence to implicate them in the anti-emetic effect of 5-HT$_3$ receptor antagonists. The reduced efficacy of 5-HT$_3$ receptor antagonists in PONV, as compared to the acute phase of chemotherapy-induced emesis, suggests that activation of a pathway containing 5-HT$_3$ receptors plays a less significant role in PONV. Based upon an understanding of the role of 5-HT and 5-HT$_3$ receptors in emesis (see above), it would be predicted that 5-HT$_3$ receptor antagonists would have the highest efficacy in abdominal and pelvic surgery when activation of the enterochromaffin cell–vagal afferent mechanism is expected to be greatest. Even in situations where 5-HT$_3$ receptors are activated by the primary emetic stimulus (e.g. abdominal surgery leading to 5-HT release) the use of drugs which do not have their emetic (or pro-emetic) effects affected by 5-HT$_3$ receptor antagonists will lead to an apparent reduction in the efficacy of the 5-HT$_3$ receptor antagonist. This has been observed in cancer patients receiving cisplatin, a 5-HT$_3$ receptor antagonist, and who were also given oral morphine (Shoji *et al.* 1999).

The transmitters most frequently implicated in the central emetic pathways are acetylcholine (acting on muscarinic M$_3$ receptors), histamine (acting on H$_1$ receptors) and dopamine (acting on D$_2$ and D$_3$ receptors). However, the site(s) at which they act are not known with any precision and they are relatively selective for particular types of emetic stimuli (e.g. H$_1$ for motion). However, blockade of one input (e.g. vestibular system, cortical arousal) may reduce the effect of activation of another input (e.g. vagal afferents) which is the primary site of action of the emetic challenge, thus providing some anti-emetic efficacy even if the anti-emetic is not targeting the primary input. This may account for the 'general' anti-emetic effects of agents, such as prochlorperazine, which have complex pharmacological actions (Rawlins *et al.* 1986). The complex pharmacology of emesis with several receptors and transmitters implicated, together with the lack of a single effective agent, has led to the proposal that 'balanced anti-emesis' should be considered for PONV (Hefferman & Rowbotham 2000). It is proposed that combinations of anti-emetic agents are used that act at different receptors. This approach has been used in chemotherapy-induced nausea and vomiting, with combinations of up to five drugs being used. This is a pragmatic approach to a difficult problem but requires care in identifying potential interactions. As mentioned above, some current agents (e.g. prochlorperazine) have effects that act on more than one receptor, but such multiple effects were not 'designed' into the original molecule. The possibility of a single agent with effects at multiple receptors has recently been reinvestigated. Yoshikawa *et al.* (2001) described an agent (AS-8112) with an antagonist action at D$_2$, D$_3$ and 5-HT$_3$ receptors and which had relatively broad-spectrum anti-emetic effects (apomorphine, morphine, cisplatin) in pre-clinical studies. This is a potentially interesting approach although clinical results on this type of compound are not available.

Preclinical studies to investigate novel approaches to anti-emesis continue. In the pig, emesis induced by lipopolysaccharides and by cisplatin can be reduced by

---

A pharmacogenetic study of 5-HT$_{3B}$ receptor gene polymorphisms in cancer patients undergoing chemotherapy and given a 5-HT$_3$ receptor antagonist to treat the emesis revealed that patients homozygous for the -100_-102delAAG deletion variant of the promoter region had more episodes of vomiting in the acute phase of emesis than patients who were not homozygous for this deletion (Tremblay *et al.* 2003). The authors comment that only a small part of the therapeutic failure of the 5-HT$_3$ receptor antagonist could be ascribed to the deletion variant. Similar studies in PONV patients would be of considerable interest especially if combined with assessment of more conventional risk factors.

cyclooxygenase (COX) inhibitors, including indomethacin and meloxicam (Girod *et al.* 2000, 2002). The efficacy of meloxicam implicates the inducible isoform COX 2 in the emetic response. These results are consistent with the anti-emetic effects of the synthetic glucocorticoids such as dexamethasone, particularly when used in combination with other anti-emetics such as 5-HT$_3$ receptor antagonists.

Cannabinoids (including marijuana) have long been known to possess anti-emetic properties but the pharmacology and site of action have not been well characterised. Two studies in ferrets (Simoneau *et al.* 2001; Van Sickle *et al.* 2001) provided evidence that the synthetic cannabinoid WIN 55, 212-2 reduced or abolished the emetic response to morphine and morphine-6-glucuronide. Evidence was presented that implicated the CB1 receptor and a site of action in the dorsal vagal complex. A CB1 receptor antagonist (AM251) potentiated the emetic response to morphine-6-glucuronide (Van Sickle *et al.* 2001) implicating endocannabinoids in the modulation of the emetic response (cf. endogenous opioid modulation: see page 14).

It must be noted that many of the clinical studies of anti-emetic efficacy were undertaken many years ago when trial design was often less rigorous than today. It would be of considerable interest to subject these studies to the type of analysis recently undertaken for the 5-HT$_3$ receptor antagonists to provide an accurate assessment of the involvement of each receptor type in PONV.

NK$_1$ receptor antagonists – the solution?

From the above discussion it is clear that identifying 'the mechanism' for PONV still lies in the future. One current approach to this and other forms of emesis where the precise mechanism is not known has been to identify 'broad-spectrum' or 'universal' anti-emetics. The ideal agent should be able to block nausea, retching and vomiting irrespective of the cause and without side-effects. In preclinical studies several receptor agonists have been shown to possess broad-spectrum anti-emetic effects. These include 5-HT$_{1A}$ (Lucot 1995), vanilloid (Andrews *et al.* 2000), and opioid (Rudd & Naylor 1995) receptor agonists. GABA$_B$ receptor agonists and cannabinoid receptor agonists also have anti-emetic effects. These agonist studies are interesting as they indicate that there are endogenous mechanisms capable of negative modulation of the emetic reflex (Figure 1.4). The site of action is unclear but the nucleus tractus solitarius and the parabrachial nucleus, which has been shown to modulate several reflexes mediated by the nucleus tractus solitarius, are likely sites. It is tempting to speculate that the intrinsic modulatory mechanism(s) is the site(s) at which at least some of the risk factors (e.g. tobacco smoking) operate. Detailed mechanistic studies of the risk factors may provide novel insights into approaches to anti-emesis.

The approach which is being most actively pursued is blockade of the neurokinin-1 (NK$_1$) receptor, the preferred ligand for the peptide neurotransmitter substance P. Pre-clinical studies have shown that a number of selective NK$_1$ receptor antagonists have broad-spectrum anti-emetic effects when studied in a range of species (Watson *et al.* 1995b; Andrews 1999b). What is meant by this is that they can markedly reduce or block retching and vomiting induced by representative stimuli acting via the vestibular system, area postrema or abdominal vagal afferents (Table 1.1).

The site of action is proposed to be in the brainstem, most likely in the nucleus tractus solitarius – the convergence point for the emetic inputs; however, the link between the nucleus tractus solitarius and the 'emetic central pattern generator' has also been proposed (Watson *et al.* 1995a; Tattersall *et al.* 1996; Fukuda *et al.* 1998). While it is clear that the NK_1 receptor antagonists can block retching and vomiting, their effect on nausea cannot easily be assessed in animal studies. Clinical studies of several NK_1 receptor antagonists (Hesketh *et al.* 1999; Navari *et al.* 1999; Rupniak & Kramer 1999; Kris *et al.* 1997; Cocquyt *et al.* 2001; Hesketh et al. 2003) in anti-cancer therapy-induced emesis are encouraging and show that this class of agent may be particularly beneficial against nausea and vomiting in the delayed phase, which is particularly resistant to conventional anti-emetics and 5-HT_3 receptor antagonists. The first member of this new class of anti-emetic agent was licensed by the F.D.A. in April 2003 and E.M.E.A in July 2003 (MK-869, Aprepitant, Emend™) for nausea and vomiting induced by highly emetic chemotherapy. Efficacy of two NK_1 receptor antagonists (CP-122, 721 and GR 205171) has been demonstrated in PONV (Gesztesi *et al.* 1998; Diemunsch *et al.* 1999). Both compounds reduced vomiting and although neither significantly reduced nausea there was a trend for GR205171 to do so when compared with placebo.

So far, clinical studies with the NK_1 receptor antagonists tested have been disappointing when compared with the preclinical studies; possible explanations for this have been discussed elsewhere (Andrews 1999b). Substance P and NK_1 receptors have been implicated in the pathophysiology of several clinically important problems and conditions (Rupniak and Kramer 1999): emesis; depression and anxiety; schizophrenia; pain (dental, osteoarthritis, neuropathic and migraine). However, limited efficacy has only been demonstrated in emesis, major depressive disorder and perhaps a weak effect in dental pain. The lack of effect in pain is surprising because of the considerable volume of evidence implicating substance P in pain pathways. This suggest that there is a fundamental problem in translating preclinical data on substance P and antagonists into clinical efficacy, a situation which contrasts markedly with 5-HT_3 receptor antagonists. It is important that the reasons are understood so that models of emesis can be refined.

Whatever the place of NK_1 receptor antagonists in the clinic, important lessons have already been learned from the study of this class of antagonist. For example, they have shown that it is possible to block emesis from three major pathways without producing any overt undesirable cardiorespiratory or behavioural effects. In addition, identification of the precise neuroanatomical site of action may point to a critical locus in the emetic pathway which is likely to have the same function in humans even if substance P and NK_1 receptors are of less importance in this region in humans. If this is the case then it could contribute to efficacy differences which may be observed between humans (and perhaps other primates) and other animals.

Table 1.1 The preclinical spectrum of the anti-emetic effects on tachykinin NK_1 receptor antagonists

Stimulus	Species	Compound
Alcohol	Suncus	CP-99,994 (Chen et al. 1997)
Apomorphine	Ferret, dog	CP-99,994 (Watson et al. 1995a)
Cisplatin (acute/delayed)	Ferret, piglet, Suncus	CP-99,994 (Watson et al. 1995a; Rudd et al. 1996); GR205171 (Grelot et al. 1998); CP122,721 (Gonsalves et al. 1996); GR-203040 (Gardner et al. 1995); PD 154075 (Saito et al. 1998)
Copper sulphate	Ferret, dog	GR203040 (Gardner et al. 1995); GR205171 (Grelot et al. 1998); CP-99,994 Watson et al. 1995a); CP-122,721 (Gonsalves et al. 1996); HSP-117 (Saito et al. 1998)
Cyclophosphamide	Ferret	GR-203040 (Gardner et al. 1995); GR205171 (Gardner et al. 1996)
Electrical vagal afferent stimulation	Ferret/dog	CP-99,994 (Watson et al. 1995a); GR205171 (Fukuda et al. 1998)
Inhaled N_2O/isoflurane	Suncus	GR205171 (Gardner & Perren 1998)
Ipecacuanha	Ferret, dog	GR203040 (Gardner et al. 1995); GR205171 (Grelot et al. 1998); CP-99,994 (Watson et al. 1995a); CP-122,721 (Gonsalves et al. 1996)
Loperamide	Ferret	CP-99,994 (Watson et al. 1995a); CP-122,721 (Gonsalves et al. 1996)
Morphine	Ferret	GR203040 (Gardner et al. 1995); GR205171 (Gardner et al. 1996); HSP-117 (Saito et al. 1998)
Motion	Suncus, cat	GR203040 (Gardner et al. 1995); GR205171; CP-99,994 (Lucot et al. 1997)
Nicotine	Suncus	CP-99,994 (Tattersall et al. 1995)
Radiation	Ferret	GR203040 (Gardner et al. 1995); CP-99,994 (Otterson et al. 1997); GR205171 (Gardner et al. 1996)
Resiniferotoxin	Suncus	CP-99,994 (Andrews and Matsuki, unpubl. observ.)
Rolipram	Ferret	CP-99,994 (Andrews and Watson, unpubl. observ)

References

Andrews, P.L.R. (1992). Physiology of nausea and vomiting. *British Journal of Anaesthesia* **69**, 2S–19S.

Andrews, P. (1993). Vomiting, a gastro-intestinal tract defensive reflex. In *Pathophysiology of the Gut and Airways. An Introduction* (ed. P. Andrews & J. Widdicombe), pp. 97–113. Portland Press, London.

Andrews, P.L.R. (1994). 5HT₃ receptor antagonists and anti-emesis. In *5HT₃ receptor antagonists* (ed. F.D. King & G.J. Sanger), pp. 255–317. CRC Press, Boca Raton, USA.

Andrews, P.L.R. (1999a). Nausea, vomiting, and the autonomic nervous system. In *Autonomic failure* (ed. C.J. Mathias & R. Bannister), pp. 126–135. Oxford University Press, Oxford.

Andrews, P.L.R. (1999b). Post-operative nausea and vomiting. In *Problems of the gastrointestinal tract in anaesthesia, the perioperative period, and intensive care* (ed. M.K. Herbert, P. Holzer & N. Roewer), pp. 267–288. Springer, Berlin-Heidelberg-New York.

Andrews, P.L.R. & Davis, C.J. (1995). The physiology of emesis induced by anticancer therapy. In *Serotonin and the scientific basis of anti-emetic therapy* (ed. D.J.M. Reynolds, P.L.R. Andrews & C.J. Davis), pp. 25–49. Oxford Clin Comm, Oxford.

Andrews, P.L.R., Bhandari, P., Garland, S., Bingham, S., Davids, C.J., Hawthorn, J., Davidson, H.I.M., Roylance, R. & Lane, S. (1990a). Does retching have a function? An experimental study in the ferret. *Pharmacodynamics and Therapeutics (Life Sciences Advances)* **9**, 135–152.

Andrews, P.L.R., Davis, C.J., Maskell, L. *et al.* (1990b). The abdominal visceral innervation and the emetic reflex: pathways, pharmacology and plasticity. *Canadian Journal of Physiology and Pharmacology* **68**, 325–345.

Andrews, P.L.R., Bhandari, P. & Davis, C.J. (1992). Plasticity and modulation of the emetic reflex. In *Mechanisms and control of emesis* (ed. A.L. Bianchi, L. Grelot, A.D. Miller & G.I. King), pp. 275–284. INSERM/John Libby Eurotext, Paris.

Apfel, C.C., Katz, M.H., Kranke, P., Goepfert, C., Papenfuss, T., Rauch, S., Heinreck, R., Greim, C-A. & Roewer, N. (2002). Volatile anaesthetics may be the main cause of early but not delayed postoperative nausea and vomiting: a randomized controlled trial of factorial design. *British Journal of Anaesthesia* **88**, 1–10.

Apfel, C.C., Kranke, P., Greim, C-A. & Roewer, N. (2001). What can be expected from risk scores for predicting post-operative nausea and vomiting? *British Journal of Anaesthesia* **86**, 822–827.

Apfel, C.C., Kranke, P., Eberhart, L.H.J., Roos, A. & Roewer, N. (2002). Comparison of predictive models for post-operative nausea and vomiting. *British Journal of Anaesthesia* **88**, 234–240.

Apfel, C.C., Läärä, E., Koivuranta, M., Greim, C-A. & Roewer, N. (1999). A simplified risk score for predicting post-operative nausea and vomiting. *Anesthesiology* **91**, 693–700.

Barann, M., Dilger, J.P., Bönisch, H., Göthert, M., Dybek, A. & Urban, B.W. (2000). Inhibition of 5-HT₃ receptors by propofol: equilibrium and kinetic measurements. *Neuropharmacology* **39**, 1064–1074.

Bentley, K.R. & Barnes, N.M. (1998). 5-hydroxytryptamine₃ (5-HT₃) receptor-mediated depolarisation of the rat isolated vagus nerve: modulation by trichloroethanol and related alcohols. *European Journal of Pharmacology* **354**, 25–31.

Chen, Y., Saito, H. & Matsuki, N. (1997). Ethanol-induced emesis in the house musk shrew, *Suncus murinus*. *Life Sciences* **60**, 253–261.

Chimbira, W. & Sweeney, B.P. (2000). The effect of smoking on post-operative nausea and vomiting. *Anaesthesia* **55**, 540–544.

Clevers, G.J., Smout, A.J.P.M., van der Schee, E.J. & Akkermans, L.M.A. (1992). Changes in gastric electrical activity in patients with severe post-operative nausea and vomiting. *Journal of Gastrointestinal Motility* **4**, 61–69.

Cocquyt, V., Van Belle, S., Reinhardt, R.R., Decramer, M.L.A., O'Brien, M., Schellens, J.H.M., Borms, M., Verbeke, L., Van Aelst, F., De Smet, M., Carides, A.D., Eldridge, K. & Gertz, B.J. (2001). Comparison of L-758, 298, a prodrug for the selective neurokinin-1 antagonists, L-754-030, with ondansetron for the prevention of cisplatin-induced emesis. *European Journal of Cancer* **37**, 835–842.

D'Acquisto, R.W., Tyson, L.B., Gralla, R.J. *et al.* (1986). The influence of a chronic high alcohol intake on chemotherapy-induced nausea and vomiting. *Proceedings of the American Society of Clinical Oncology* **5**, 257.

Desbiens, N.A., Mueller-Rizner, N., Connors, A-F. & Wenger, N.S. (1997). The relationship of nausea and dyspnea to pain in seriously ill patients. *Pain* **71**, 149–156.

Diemunsch, P., Schoeffler, P., Bryssine, B., Cheli-Muller, L.E., Lees, J., McQuade, B.A. & Spraggs, C.F. (1999). Antiemetic activity of the NK_1 receptor antagonist GR205171 in the treatment of established post-operative nausea and vomiting after major gynaecological surgery. *British Journal of Anaesthesia* **82**, 274–276.

Eden, D. & Zuk, Y. (1995). Seasickness as a self-fulfilling prophecy: raising self-efficacy to boost performance at sea. *Journal of Applied Psychology* **80**, 628–635.

Fredrikson, M., Hursti, T., Fürst, C.J., Steinbeck, G., Börjeson, S. & Wikblom, M. (1992) Nausea in cancer chemotherapy is inversely related to urinary cortisol excretion. *British Journal of Cancer* **65**, 779–780.

Fredrikson, M., Hursti, T., Steinbeck, G., Fürst, C.J., Börjeson, S. & Peterson, C. (1994). Delayed chemotherapy-induced nausea is augmented by high levels of endogenous noradrenaline. *British Journal of Cancer* **70**, 642–645.

Fukuda, H. & Koga, T. (1993). Hypercapnia and hypoxia which developed during retching participate in the transition from retching to expulsion in dogs. *Neuroscience Research* **17**, 205–215.

Fukuda, H., Koga, T., Furukawa, N., Nakamura, E. & Shiroshita, Y. (1998). The tachykinin NK_1 receptor antagonist GR205171 prevents vagal stimulation-induced retching but not neuronal transmission from emetic vagal afferents to solitary nucleus neurons in dogs. *Brain Research* **802**, 221–231.

Gadsby, R., Barnie-Adshead, A.M. & Jagger, C. (1997). Pregnancy nausea related to women's obstetric and personal histories. *Gynecology and Obstetric Investigation* **43**, 108–111.

Gardner, C. & Perren, M. (1998). Inhibition of anaesthetic-induced emesis by a NK_1 or $5\text{-}HT_3$ receptor antagonist in the house musk shrew, *Suncus murinus. Neuropharmacology* **37**, 1643–1644.

Gardner, C.J., Twissell, D.J., Dale, T.J., Gale, J.D., Jordan, C.C., Kilpatrick, G.H., Bountra, C. & Ward, P. (1995). The broad-spectrum anti-emetic activity of the novel non-peptide tachykinin NK_1 receptor antagonist GR203040. *British Journal of Pharmacology* **116**, 3158–3163.

Gardner, C.J., Armour, D.R., Beattie, D.T., Gale, J.D., Hawcock, A.B., Kilpatrick, G.J., Twissell, D.J. & Ward, P. (1996). GR205171: a novel antagonist with high affinity for the tachykinin NK_1 receptor, and potent broad-spectrum anti-emetic activity. *Regulatory Peptides* **65**, 45–53.

Gesztesi, Z.S., Song, D. & White, P.F. (1998). Comparison of a new NK-1 antagonist (CP122,721). to ondansetron in the prevention of postoperative nausea and vomiting. *Anesthesia and Analgesia* **86**, S32.

Girod, V., Bouvier, M. & Grélot, L. (2000) Characterization of lipopolysaccharide-induced emesis in conscious piglets: effects of cervical vagotomy, cyclooxygenase inhibitors and a 5-HT$_3$ receptor antagonist. *Neuropharmacology* **39**, 2329–2335.

Girod, V., Dapzol, J., Bouvier, M. & Grélot, L. (2002) The COX inhibitors indomethacin and meloxicam exhibit anti-emetic activity against cisplatin-induced emesis in piglets. *Neuropharmacology* **42**, 428–436.

Gonsalves, S., Watson & Ashton, C. (1996). Broad-spectrum antiemetic effects of CP-122,721, a tachykinin NK$_1$ receptor antagonist, in ferrets. *European Journal of Pharmacology* **305**, 181–185.

Greenland, S., Satterfield, M.H. & Lanes, S.F. (1998). A meta-analysis to assess the incidence of adverse effects associated with the transdermal nicotine patch. *Drug Safety* **18**, 297–308.

Grelot, L. & Miller, A.D. (1996). Neural control of respiratory muscle activation during vomiting. In *Neural control of respiratory muscles* (ed. A.D. Miller, A.L. Bianchi & B.P. Bishop), pp. 239–248. CRC Press Inc, Boca Raton, USA.

Grelot, L., Dapzol, J., Esteve, E., Frugiere, A., Bianchi, A.L., Sheldrick, R.L.G., Gardner, C.J. & Ward, P. (1998). Potent inhibition of both the acute and delayed emetic responses to cisplatin in piglets treated with GR205171, a novel highly selective tachykinin NK$_1$ receptor antagonist, in ferrets. *European Journal of Pharmacology* **305**, 181–185.

Grundy, D. & Scratcherd, T. (1989). Sensory afferents from the gastrointestinal tract. In *Handbook of physiology*, Section 6: *The gastrointestinal system*; Vol 1. *Motility and circulation*; Part 1 (ed. J.D. Wood), pp. 593–620. American Physiology Society, Bethesda, USA.

Hefferman, A.M. & Rowbotham, D.J. (2000). Post-operative nausea and vomiting – time for balanced antiemesis? *British Journal of Anaesthesia* **85**, 675–677.

Herbert, M.K., Holzer, P. & Roewer, N. (ed.) (1999). *Problems of the gastrointestinal tract in anaesthesia, the perioperative period, and intensive care.* Springer, Berlin-Heidelberg-New York.

Hesketh, P.J., Gralla, R.J., Webb, R.T., Ueno, W., DelPrete, S., Bachinsky, M.E., Dirlam, N.L., Stack, C.B. & Silberman, S.L. (1999). Randomized Phase II study of the neurokinin 1 receptor antagonist CJ-11,974 in the control of cisplatin-induced emesis. *Journal of Clinical Oncology* **17**, 338–343.

Hesketh, P.J., Van Belle, S., Aapro, M., Tattersall, F.D., Naylor, R.J., Hargreaves, R., Carides, A.D., Evans, J.K. & Horgan, K.J. (2003). Differential involvement of neurotransmitters through the time course of cisplatin-induced emesis as revealed by therapy with specific receptor antagonists. *European Journal of Cancer* **39**, 1074–1080.

Hillsley, K. & Grundy, D. (1998). Sensitivity to 5-hydroxytryptamine in different afferent sub-populations within mesenteric nerves supplying the rat jejunum. *Journal of Physiology* **509**, 717–727.

Hursti, T.J., Fredrikson, M., Steineck, G., Börjeson, S., Fürst, C.J. & Peterson, C. (1993). Endogenous cortisol exerts antiemetic effect similar to that of exogenous corticosteroids. *British Journal of Cancer* **68**, 112–114.

Iovino, P., Azpiroz, F., Domingo, E. & Malagelada, J-R. (1995). The sympathetic nervous system modulates perception and reflex responses to gut distention in humans. *Gastroenterology* **108**, 680–686.

Isaacs, B. (1957). The influence of head and body position on the emetic action of apomorphine in man. *Clinical Science* **16**, 215–221.

Koch, K.L. (1993). Motion sickness. In *The handbook of nausea and vomiting* (ed. M Sleisenger), pp.43–60. Parthenon Publishing Group, New York, USA.

Koch, K.L. (1995). Approach to the patient with nausea and vomiting. In *Textbook of gastro-enterology* 2nd edn (ed. T Yamada), pp. 731–49. J.B. Lippincott Co, Philadelphia, USA.

Koch, K.L. (1997). A noxious trio – nausea, gastric dysrhythmias and vasopressin. *Neurogastroenterology and Motility* **9**, 141–142.

Koga, T. & Fukuda, H. (1990). Characteristic behavior of the respiratory muscles, esophagus, and external anal and urethral sphincters during straining, retching, and vomiting in the decerebrate dog. *Japanese Journal of Physiology* **40**, 789–807.

Koga, T., Qu, R. & Fukuda, H. (1998). The central pattern generator for vomiting may exist in the reticular area dorsomedial to the retrofacial nucleus in dogs. *Experimental Brain Research* **118**, 139–147.

Kranke, P., Apfel, C.C., Papenfuss, T., Meyer, F., Sefrin, P. & Roewer, N. (1998). Influence of low-dose opioids for induction of inhalational anaesthesia on postoperative nausea and vomiting. *Anästhesiologie Intensivmedizin Notfallmedizin Schmerztherapie* **9**, 616S.

Kris, M.G., Radford, J., Pizzo, B.A. *et al.* (1997). Control of emesis following cisplatin by CP-122,721, a selective NK_1 receptor antagonist. *Journal of the National Cancer Institutes* **89**, 817–818.

Lang, I.M. (1990). Digestive tract motor correlates of vomiting and nausea. *Canadian Journal of Physiology and Pharmacology* **68**, 242–253.

Lang, I.M., Sarna, S.K. & Dodds, W.J. (1993). Pharyngeal, esophageal, and proximal gastric responses associated with vomiting. *American Journal of Physiology* **265**, G963–G972.

Leslie, R.A. & Reynolds, D.J.M. (1991). The area postrema and vomiting, how important is serotonin? In *Current aspects of the neurosciences* (ed. N.N. Osborne) pp. 79–101. Macmillan, Basingstoke.

Leslie, R.A. & Reynolds, D.J.M. (1992). Functional anatomy of the emetic circuitry in the brainstem. In *Mechanisms and control of emesis* (ed. AL Bianchi, L Grelot, AD Miller & GL King), pp. 19–27. Colloque INSERM/John Libbey Eurotext Ltd, Paris, Montrouge, France.

Lindstrom, P.A. & Brizzee, K.R. (1962). Relief of intractable vomiting from surgical lesions in the area postrema. *Journal of Neurosurgery* **19**, 228–236.

Lucot, J.B. (1995). $5\text{-}HT_{1A}$ receptor agonists as anti-emetics. In *Serotonin and the scientific basis of anti-emetic therapy* (ed. DJM Reynolds, PLR Andrews & CJ Davis) pp. 222–227. Oxford Clinical Communications, Oxford.

Lucot, J.B., Obach, R.S., McLean, S. & Watson, J.W. (1997). The effect of CP-99,994 on the responses to provocative motion in the cat. *British Journal of Pharmacology* **120**, 116–120.

Makale, M.T. & King, G.L. (1993). Plasticity of autonomic control of emesis in irradiated ferrets. *American Journal of Physiology* **265**, R1092–R1099.

Matsuki, N., Wang, C-H., Okada, F., Tamura, M., Ikegaya, Y., Lin, S-C., Hsu, Y-N., Chaung, L-J., Chen, S-J. & Saito, H. (1997). Male/female differences in drug-induced emesis and motion sickness in *Suncus murinus*. *Pharmacology Biochemistry and Behaviour* **57**, 721–725.

Miller, A.D., Rowley, H.A., Roberts, T.P.L. & Kucharczyk, J. (1996). Human cortical activity during vestibular- and drug-induced nausea detected using MSI. *Annals of the New York Academy of Sciences* **781**, 670–672.

Minami, M., Endo, T., Nemoto, M., Hamaue, N., Hirafuji, M., Monama, Y., Yajima, T., Yoshioka, M. & Saito, H. (1995). The physiology of emesis induced by anticancer therapy. In *Serotonin and the scientific basis of anti-emetic therapy* (ed. D.J.M. Reynolds, P.L.R. Andrews & C.J. Davis) pp.68–83. Oxford Clinical Communications, Oxford.

Morrow, G.R., Roscoe, J.A., Kirshner, J.J., Hynes, H.E. & Rosenbluth, R.J. (1998). Anticipatory nausea and vomiting in the era of $5\text{-}HT_3$ antiemetics. *Supportive Care in Cancer* **6**, 244–247.

Navari, R.M., Reinhardt, R.R., Gralla, R.J., Kris, M.G., Hesketh, P.J., Khojasteh, A., Kindler, H., Grote, T.H., Pendergrass, K., Grunberg, S.M., Carides, A.D. & Gertz, B.J. (1999). Reduction of cisplatin-induced emesis by a selective neurokinin-1 receptor antagonist. *New England Journal of Medicine* **340**, 190–195.

Nussey, S.S., Hawthorn, J., Page, S.R., Ang, V.T.Y. & Jenkins, J.S. (1988). Responses of plasma oxytocin and arginine vasopressin to nausea induced by apomorphine and ipecacuanha. *Clinical Endocrinology* **28**, 297–304.

Otterson, M.F., Leming, S.C. & Moulder, J.E. (1997). Central NK1 receptors mediate radiation induced emesis. *Gastroenterology* **112**, A801.

Palazzo, M.G.A. & Strunin, L. (1984). Anaesthesia and emesis. I: Etiology. *Canadian Anaesthesia Society Journal* **31**, 178–187.

Parker, R.M.C., Bentley, K.R. & Barnes, N.M. (1996). Allosteric modulation of 5-HT$_3$ receptors: focus on alcohols and anaesthetic agents. *Trends in Pharmacological Science* **17**, 95–99.

Peters, J.A. & Lambert, J.J. (1997). Anesthetics in a bind? *Trends in Pharmacological Science* **18**, 454–455.

Racke, K. & Schwoerer, H. (1991). Regulation of serotonin release from the intestinal mucosa. *Pharmacology Research* **23**, 13–25.

Rawlins, M.D., Taylor, W.B. & Bateman, D.N. (1986). Rational approaches to therapy for nausea and vomiting: two common solutions. In *Nausea and vomiting: mechanisms and treatment* (ed. C.J. Davis, Lake-Bakaar & D.G. Grahame-Smith), pp. 167–171. Springer-Verlag, Berlin.

Rudd, J.A. & Naylor, R.J. (1995). Opioid receptor involvement in emesis and anti-emesis. In *Serotonin and the scientific basis of anti-emetic therapy* (ed. D.J.M. Reynolds, P.L.R. Andrews & C.J. Davis) pp. 208–21. Oxford Clinical Communications, Oxford.

Rudd, J.A., Cheng, C.H.K., Naylor, R.J., Ngan, M.P. & Wai, M.K. (1999). Modulation of emesis by fentanyl and opioid receptor antagonists in *Suncus murinus* (house musk shrew). *European Journal of Pharmacology* **374**, 77–84.

Rudd, J.A., Jordan, C.C. & Naylor, R.J. (1996). The action of the NK$_1$ tachykinin receptor antagonist, CP 99,994 in antagonizing the acute and delayed emesis induced by cisplatin in the ferret. *British Journal of Pharmacology* **119**, 931–936.

Rupniak, N.M.J. & Kramer, M.S. (1999). Discovery of the antidepressant and anti-emetic efficacy of substance P receptor (NK$_1$) antagonists. *Trends in Pharmacological Science* **20**, 485–490.

Saito, R., Suehiro, Y., Ariumi, H., Migita, K., Hori, N., Hashiguchi, T., Sakai, M., Saeki, M., Takano, Y. & Kamiya, H-O. (1998). Anti-emetic effects of a novel NK-1 receptor antagonist HSP-117 in ferrets. *Neuroscience Letters* **254**, 169–172.

Sanger, G.J. & Andrews, P.L.R. (2001). Emesis. In *Drug Therapy for Gastrointestinal and Liver Diseases* (eds. M.J.G. Farthing & A.B. Ballinger) pp. 44–61. Martin Dunitz, London, UK.

Sem-Jacobsen, C.W. (1968). *Depth electrographic stimulation of the human brain and behavior.* Thomas, Springfield (Ill.), USA.

Shoji, A., Toda, M., Suzuki, K., Takahashi, H., Takahashi, K., Yoshiike, Y., Ogura, T., Watanuki Y., Nishiyama, H. & Odagiri, S. (1999). Insufficient effectiveness of 5-hydroxytryptamine-3 receptor antagonists due to oral morphine administration in patients with cisplatin-induced emesis. *Journal of Clinical Oncology* **17**, 1926–1930.

Singh, L., Field, M.J., Hughes, J., Kuo, B-S., Suman-Chauhan, N., Tuladhar, B.R., Wright, D.S. & Naylor, R.J. (1997). The tachykinin NK$_1$ receptor antagonist PD 154075 blocks cisplatin-induced delayed emesis in the ferret. *European Journal of Pharmacology* **321**, 209–216.

Simoneau, I.I., Hamza, M.S., Mata, H.P., Siegel, E.M., Vanderah, T.W., Porreca, F., Makriyannis, A. & Malan, T.P. (2001). The cannabinoid agonist WIN55,212-2 suppresses opioid-induced emesis in ferrets. *Anaesthesiology* **94**, 882–887.

Tannahill, R. (1996). *Flesh and blood. A history of the cannibal complex.* Abacus, London.

Tattersall, F.D., Rycroft, W., Marmont, N., Cascieri, M., Hill, R.G. & Hargreaves, R.J. (1995). Enantiospecific inhibition of emesis induced by nicotine in the house musk shrew (*Suncus murinus*) by the Neurokinin$_1$ (NK$_1$) receptor antagonist CP-99,994. *Neuropharmacology* **34**, 1697–1699.

Tattersall, F.D., Rycroft, W., Francis, B., Pearce, D., Merchant, K., MacLeod, A.M., Ladduwahetty, T., Keown, L., Swain, C., Baker, R., Cascieri, M., Ber, E., Metzger, J., MacIntyre, D.E., Hill, R.G. & Hargreaves, R.J. (1996). Tachykinin NK$_1$ receptor antagonists act centrally to inhibit emesis induced by the chemotherapeutic agent cisplatin in ferrets. *Neuropharmacology* **35**, 1121–1129.

Thompson, P.I., Bingham, S., Andrews, P.L.R., Patel, N., Joel, S.P. & Slevin, M.L. (1992). Morphine 6-glucuronide: a metabolite of morphine with greater emetic potency than morphine in the ferret. *British Journal of Pharmacology* **106**, 3–8.

Tremblay, P.B., Kaiser, R., Sezer, O., Roler, N., Schelenz, C., Possinger, K., Roots, I. & Brockmoller, J. (2003). Variations in the 5-HT$_{3B}$ receptor gene as predictors of the efficacy of anti-emetic treatment in cancer patients. *Journal of Clinical Oncology* **21**, 2147–2155.

Van Sickle, M.D., Oland, L.D., Ho, W., Hillard, C.J., Mackie, K., Davison, J.S. & Sharkey, K.A. (2001). Cannabinoids inhibit emesis through CB1 receptors in the brainstem of the ferret. *Gastroenterology* **121**, 767–774.

Watcha, M.F. & White, P.F. (1992). Postoperative nausea and vomiting – its etiology, treatment and prevention. *Anesthesiology* **77**, 162–184.

Watson, J.W., Gonsalves, S.F., Fossa, A.A., McLean, S., Seeger, T., Obach, S. & Andrews, P.L.R. (1995a). The anti-emetic effects of CP-99,994 in the ferret and the dog: role of the NK$_1$ receptor. *British Journal of Pharmacology* **115**, 84–94.

Watson, J.W., Nagahisa, A., Lucot, J.B. & Andrews, P.L.R. (1995b). The tachykinins and emesis: towards complete control? In *Serotonin and the scientific basis of anti-emetic therapy* (ed. DJM Reynolds, PLR Andrews & CJ Davis) pp. 233–238. Oxford Clinical Communications, Oxford.

Whitwam, J.G., Morgan, M., Owen, J.R., Goolden, A.W.G., Spiers, A.S.D., Goldman, J.M. & Gordon-Smith, E.C. (1978). General anaesthesia for high-dose total body irradiation. *Lancet* **i**, 128–129.

Xu, L.H., Koch, K.L., Summy-Long, J., Stern, R.M., Seaton, J.F., Harrison, T.S., Demers, L.M. & Bingaman, S. (1993). Hypothalamic and gastric myoelectrical responses during vection-induced nausea in healthy Chinese subjects. *American Journal of Physiology* **265**, E578–E584.

Yoshikawa, T., Yoshida, N. & Oka, M. (2001). The broad-spectrum anti-emetic activity of AS-8112, a novel dopamine D$_2$, D$_3$ and 5-HT$_3$ receptors antagonist. *British Journal of Pharmacology* **133**, 253–260.

Chapter 2

Epidemiological aspects of post-operative nausea and vomiting and assessment of risk

R.A. Struthers and J.R. Sneyd

Introduction

Post-operative nausea and vomiting (PONV) were first described in 1848 by John Snow (Snow 1848), within 18 months of the introduction of anaesthesia to Britain. The belief that anaesthetics alone were responsible for most cases of PONV persisted until 1916 when Flagg reported that post-operative vomiting may result from other causes including pain, ovarian surgery, reflex responses and opioids (Flagg 1916). In 1960 Bellville and colleagues suggested that choice of anaesthetic agent, the type of surgery and administration of anti-emetic were likely to influence the incidence and severity of PONV (Bellville *et al.* 1960).

Nausea and vomiting may prolong hospital stay (Chung & Mezei 1999) and necessitate the use of anti-emetic medication with corresponding costs and side effects. Studies into patients' experiences of anaesthesia and surgery suggest that avoidance of PONV is a high priority (Macario *et al.* 1999; Myles *et al.* 2000; Jenkins *et al.* 2001; Gan *et al.* 2001).

The incidence of PONV in adults is approximately 25%, ranging from 6% to 70% in published series (Honkavaara *et al.* 1991; Koivuranta *et al.* 1997; Bacic *et al.* 1998; Apfel *et al.* 1999; Chimbira & Sweeney 2000). Review of the literature on individual factors contributing to PONV is complicated by lack of standardisation of the definitions of 'nausea' and 'vomiting' and frequently by the failure to control other factors that may contribute to PONV. Patients may experience PONV up to 36 hours after surgery, necessitating a suitable time-course for follow-up. Research into PONV is further complicated by variability both within an individual and between individuals, and the lack of a commonly accepted animal model.

The epidemiological factors of PONV can be divided into patient, surgical and anaesthetic factors.

Patient factors

Age and sex

In children the risk of PONV is commonly reported as almost twice that for adults (Vance *et al.* 1973; Cohen *et al.* 1990). However, few data exist to compare the incidence under controlled circumstances, i.e. adults and children undergoing similar procedures with the same anaesthetic technique. There is an equal distribution of PONV between boys and girls until puberty (Vance *et al.* 1973; Rowley & Brown 1982). Adult women are two to three times more likely to suffer from PONV than men (Palazzo & Evans 1993; Apfel *et al.* 1999; Sinclair *et al.* 1999) until after the menopause when rates equalise (Purkis 1964). In ambulatory patients it would appear that PONV decreases with age (Chung *et al.* 1999).

Phase of menstrual cycle

An influence of the menstrual cycle on PONV has been suspected for some time but findings have been conflicting. In 1961 Bellville reported that in adult females the highest incidence of PONV occurred during the third and fourth weeks of the menstrual cycle (Bellville 1961). Honkavaara found PONV to be more common during the luteal phase (days 20–24), compared with the follicular phase (days 8–12) and the premenstrual and menstrual phase (days 25–26) (Honkavaara *et al.* 1991) and in another *post hoc* study they showed increased PONV in the periovulatory days (days 11–24) (Honkavaara *et al.* 1996). Beattie found conflicting results – that PONV was highest in the first eight days of the cycle and lowest on days 18–20 (Beattie *et al.* 1991). Bacic found that the incidence was highest in the periovulatory and premenstrual phases of the cycle (Bacic *et al.* 1998) whereas Konvalinka found more PONV in menstruating women (Konvalinka 1999). In addition, studies have found that women with irregular cycles – who may make up 25% of the surgical population – had a higher incidence of PONV than those with regular cycles (Harmon *et al.* 2000) and that women in the same phase of the cycle are more likely to vomit if they have higher oestrogen levels (Linbland *et al.* 1990).

Potential explanations for these conflicting findings may include deficiencies in study design – including recall bias in the women giving incorrect information as to phase of the cycle. PONV may also be related to hormonal interactions not directly related to the menstrual cycle.

Previous PONV

In 1964 Purkis reported that the incidence of PONV was three times greater in patients with previous PONV (Purkis 1964). This finding has been confirmed in subsequent studies and a history of PONV has been incorporated as an independent variable into models trying to predict PONV (Palazzo & Evans 1993; Koivuranta *et al.* 1997; Apfel *et al.* 1999; Sinclair *et al.* 1999).

Motion Sickness

Palazzo (Palazzo & Evans 1993) and Toner (Toner *et al.* 1996) confirmed an association between a history of motion sickness and PONV. Subsequent scoring systems have incorporated motion sickness as an independent variable (Koivuranta *et al.* 1997; Sinclair *et al.* 1999) or in combination with previous PONV (Apfel *et al.* 1999).

Patient transport may trigger emesis in those prone to motion sickness (see Kamath *et al.* 1990) and this factor may not be controlled in clinical trials.

Smoking

Smoking appears to be protective against PONV. Smoking was studied independently of other risk factors by Chimbira and Sweeny. In their study of 327 day-case knee arthroscopies, 15% of non-smokers suffered from PONV compared with 6% of smokers (Chimbira & Sweeney 2000). Again, predictive models by Koivuranta (Koivuranta *et al.* 1997), Sinclair (Sinclair *et al.* 1999), and Apfel (Apfel *et al.* 1999) have used non-smoking status as an independent risk factor for PONV whereas the Palazzo model does not (Palazzo & Evans 1993).

Obesity

Although some authorities have suggested an excess of PONV in obese patients (Palazzo & Strunin 1984; Watcha & White 1992), this association is not generally accepted. Muir studied 780 patients and found no relation between body mass index (BMI) and the incidence of PONV (Muir *et al.* 1987). A systematic review has suggested that there is no link between BMI and PONV (Kranke *et al.* 2001). The predictive equation of Palazzo did not include any independent term for BMI or weight (Palazzo & Evans 1993) and subsequent predictive models have not found BMI to be a factor in PONV (Koivuranta *et al.* 1997; Apfel *et al.* 1999; Sinclair *et al.* 1999).

Surgical factors

Nature of operation

Since 1916, when Flagg suggested an association between ovarian surgery and PONV (Flagg 1916), wide discrepancies in incidences of PONV have been reported in association with the surgery undertaken (Rowley & Brown 1982; Pataky *et al.* 1988).

Children

In children, the procedure most commonly associated with the highest incidence of PONV is correction of squints, where the incidence is between 40% and 88% in children older than 2 years (Lerman *et al.* 1986; van den Berg *et al.* 1987; Warner *et al.* 1988; van den Berg *et al.* 1989; Lin *et al.* 1992; Schlager *et al.* 2000). The use of newer anti-emetics and combinations of drugs has lead to published vomiting rates as low as 5% (Splinter & Rhine 1998; Splinter 2001). No correlation has been found demonstrated between the number of extra-ocular muscles repaired and the incidence of PONV (Smith & Manford 1974; Lerman *et al.* 1986).

After adeno-tonsillectomy the incidence of post-operative vomiting is 23–78% (Rowley & Brown 1982; Puttick & Van der Walt 1987; Holt *et al.* 2000; Aouad *et al.* 2001; Mukherjee *et al.* 2001) and may be attributed to three mechanisms: (i) blood in the upper gastrointestinal tract; (ii) stimulation of trigeminal nerve afferents during surgery; and (iii) the administration of perioperative opioids.

Adults

In adults, abdominal, gynaecological and ear, nose and throat surgery account for the highest incidence of PONV. When different studies have examined rates of PONV, however, they have found no surgery with consistently high rates of PONV that can be used as a predictive variable for models of PONV. Of the models already mentioned, only Sinclair uses type of surgery to try to predict PONV, having found plastic and orthopaedic surgery to have a higher rate of PONV (Sinclair *et al.* 1999). Explanations for PONV in open abdominal and laparoscopic surgery have included gut ischaemia causing the release of serotonin and subsequent nausea.

Length of operation

Several investigations have reported on the relation between the duration of surgery and PONV but the results are conflicting and recent data scanty. Early studies reported an almost 3-fold increase after longer procedures (Bellville *et al.* 1960) whereas others found no correlation (Gold 1969). More recently Sinclair *et al.* (1999) found a direct correlation between duration of surgery of up to 3 hours duration and risk of PONV. Koivuranta (Koivuranta *et al.* 1997) found an association with surgery lasting over 60 minutes. Both included it in their predictive models whereas the other models previously discussed (Palazzo & Evans 1993; Apfel *et al.* 1999) did not. A more recent study by Apfel suggested that the risk of PONV was increased by 1.4 times for every hour of anaesthesia (Apfel *et al.* 2002).

Anaesthetic factors

Anaesthetist

It has been 'known' for many years that the experienced anaesthetist has fewer patients who suffer from PONV than the inexperienced (Rubin & Metz-Rubin 1951; Bellville *et al.* 1960). It was suggested that this was because the inexperienced anaesthetist tended to maintain the patient at a deeper level of anaesthesia (Bellville 1961).This has been supported by recent work using processed EEG monitoring to monitor depth of anaesthesia, which showed less early PONV in those where the anaesthetic was guided by the EEG (Nelskyla *et al.* 2001).

In addition, manual inflation of the lungs by an inexperienced anaesthetist using a face mask before tracheal intubation was associated with a higher incidence of PONV than when the anaesthetist was experienced (Hovorka *et al.* 1990). This may be due to inadvertent insufflation of the stomach with air. Other workers have also implicated mask ventilation as a cause of PONV (Dent *et al.* 1955) and found greater PONV when the laryngeal mask airway (LMA) was used for intermittent positive pressure ventilation rather than an endotracheal tube (Swann *et al.* 1993). However, in a study where half of the 201 subjects had their stomach aspirated at the end of surgery there was no difference in rates of PONV (Hovorka *et al.* 1990) and a further study of 265 patients showed increased rates of late PONV if the stomach was suctioned (Trepanier & Isabel 1993).

Premedication

Centrally acting anti-cholinergics such as hyoscine and atropine may reduce the incidence of PONV (Mirakhur 1991) whereas glycopyrrolate, which does not cross the blood–brain barrier, does not (Salmenpera *et al.* 1992). The role of anxiolytic premedication is unclear. The use of temazepam in adults may reduce PONV (Kamath *et al.* 1990). In children PONV has been shown to be unrelated to pre-operative anxiety (Wang & Kain 2000) but clonidine as a sedative premedication has been shown to be superior to diazepam in reducing PONV (Mikawa *et al.* 1995; Handa & Fujii 2001).

Anaesthetic agents

The induction agents methohexitone and etomidate are associated with a significant increase in PONV compared with sodium thiopentone and propofol (Clarke 1984).

Many studies have reported a reduced incidence of PONV when anaesthesia was induced or maintained with propofol; however, individual studies often lack statistical power. Meta-analysis is a statistical process whereby data from multiple studies is combined to yield an overall summary statistic (Chalmers & Altman 1995). For meta-analysis to be useful it is important for all relevant studies to be identified and for heterogeneity between studies to be investigated. Publication bias, the tendency for studies with positive results to achieve priority in publication over those with negative or neutral findings, is an important source of heterogeneity. All data from meta-analysis must therefore be viewed with appropriate caution. Three groups have used meta-analysis to compare the incidence of nausea and vomiting after inhalational and intravenous maintenance of anaesthesia. Jobalia and Mathieu (1994) relied exclusively on a MEDLINE search and identified 28 studies covering 1116 patients who were randomised to maintenance of anaesthesia with propofol or an inhalational agent. They reported that the odds ratios for PONV after maintenance with propofol were 0.29, 0.25 and 0.29 for vomiting, nausea and 'nausea and vomiting' respectively. Tramer *et al.* (1997b) undertook a meta-analysis of 84 studies covering 6069 patients randomised to intravenous induction or maintenance of anaesthesia with propofol, or 'other anaesthetics' which included inhalational anaesthesia as well as propanidid, midazolam or alphaxolone. They found that use of propofol as the induction agent was associated with a reduced risk of early nausea and vomiting (odds ratios of 0.45 and 0.47, respectively).When propofol was also used to maintain anaesthesia, the odds ratios were 0.34 and 0.25 for nausea and vomiting respectively within the first 6 hours after anaesthesia and 0.36 and 0.55 respectively beyond 6 hours. They also calculated the 'number-needed-to-treat' (Cook & Sackett 1995), i.e. the number of patients who would need to be given propofol anaesthesia to avoid one case of nausea or vomiting as 4.7 and 4.9 respectively. A meta-analysis by Sneyd *et al.* (1998) reviewed 96 studies. Many of these studies had multiple treatment arms and after excluding the least appropriate compactor groups, data from 5214 patients were analysed. The odds ratios for nausea, vomiting and 'nausea or vomiting' were 0.38, 0.27 and 0.37, respectively, yielding a number-needed-to-treat of 8.1, 7.1 and 6.6 respectively. Sub-group analysis suggested that type of surgery, opioid usage, patient age and nitrous oxide usage did not affect the odds ratios obtained. When propofol was compared with sevoflurane and desflurane the findings were similar to comparisons with older agents, i.e. the newer inhalational anaesthetic agents do not appear to reduce PONV (Sneyd *et al.* 1998).

Although no large randomised study has been done to definitively address the benefits of intravenous anaesthesia, a Phase IV prospective study of 25,981 patients in 1772 hospitals revealed a low incidence (1.9%) of PONV after propofol anaesthesia (McLeskey *et al.* 1993).

The use of propofol as a true anti-emetic in subhypnotic doses is less well defined, with studies showing its efficacy at close to sedative doses (Kim *et al.* 2000) and no effect at lower doses (Montgomery *et al.* 1996; Bree *et al.* 1998).

The association between induction and maintenance of anaesthesia with propofol and a reduced risk of PONV is now well established. However, the relative utility of this approach and other PONV reduction strategies has not been critically compared. Critics of intravenous anaesthesia point to the number-needed-to-treat and question whether this technique is a cost-effective method of reducing PONV (Tramer *et al.* 1997a, b). Crucially, the interaction between different components of PONV remains uncertain. Thus nitrous oxide alone is certainly emetogenic but its contribution may be small relative to other factors when it is used a component of a balanced anaesthetic (Hovorka *et al.* 1989; Sneyd *et al.* 1998).

Neuromuscular blocking and reversal agents

The neuromuscular blocking agents in current use have not been shown to have an effect on PONV. It was thought that the use of neostigmine to reverse muscle paralysis was strongly correlated with PONV (King *et al.* 1988). However, recent work suggests this is not the case (Hovorka *et al.* 1997; Nelskyla *et al.* 1998).

Peri-operative opioids

All agents that act at the μ-opioid receptor appear to cause nausea and vomiting and attempts to separate this effect from analgesic efficacy have been unsuccessful. The role of opioids in PONV is unclear as intravenous techniques generally include an opioid but have a low incidence of PONV (Sneyd *et al.* 1998). These data suggest that the contribution of anaesthetic drugs to PONV is dominated by the choice of maintenance agent with opioids acting as a less important factor.

Maintenance of anaesthesia with remifentanil subjects the patient to a period intense μ-opioid receptor stimulation yet PONV is no more common than with other opioids which would normally be used at a much lower dose (after adjustment for potency). Perhaps the influence of opioids on PONV is determined by their presence in the conscious rather than the unconscious patient? In a recent study looking at risk factors for PONV, post-operative opioids were associated with an increased risk whereas intraoperative opioids were not (Apfel *et al.* 2002).

Anaesthetic techniques

Spinal anaesthesia

In a prospective study of 952 patients undergoing spinal anaesthesia, the overall incidence of nausea was 18% and vomiting 7% (Carpenter *et al.* 1992). The addition of adrenaline to the local anaesthetic, blocks with a sensory level higher than the fifth thoracic dermatome, and hypotension were associated with the greatest risk of PONV. The use of ephedrine to minimise hypotension (Datta *et al.* 1982) and administration of 100% oxygen (Ratra *et al.* 1972) have been reported to reduce intra-operative nausea and vomiting. In a more recent study the administration of 20 ml/kg of Ringers lactate at the time of spinal anaesthetic did not reduce hypotension compared to giving the same fluid bolus 20 minutes before surgery but it did reduce intraoperative nausea, vomiting and faintness (Mojica *et al.* 2002). PONV was not considered.

Regional techniques

When neural block of limbs with local anaesthetics was compared with spinal anaesthesia, the incidence of PONV was reduced for 24 hours (Dent *et al.* 1955; Bonica *et al.* 1958). This may reflect the different haemodynamic consequences of the two techniques. More generally, regional techniques may reduce patient exposure to opiates, general anaesthetics and haemodynamic fluctuations – all of which may be related to increased PONV (D'Alessio *et al.* 1995; Coveney *et al.* 1998).

Oxygenation

The use of high inspired oxygen to reduce intraoperative nausea and vomiting was described some time ago in spinal anaesthesia (Ratra *et al.* 1972). More recently, subgroup analysis of a large study where half of the patients were given 80% oxygen balance nitrogen vs. 30% oxygen both during surgery and for 2 hours afterwards showed PONV rates of 17% and 30% respectively (Greif *et al.* 1999). There appeared to be no differences in pulmonary complications. The authors then set out to study the same oxygen ratios in gynaecological laparoscopies and showed that the use of 80% oxygen was at least as efficacious as ondansetron 8 mg (Goll *et al.* 2001). The anti-emetic properties of oxygen were further studied recently in elderly patients being transported to hospital after minor trauma. Those who were given oxygen at 10 L/min had significantly less nausea and vomiting compared with those given air

et al. 2002). It has been suggested that high levels of oxygen
nine release and that transient ischaemia may cause 5-HT release
er of which might be related to PONV.

...ydration

In a study of day-case gynaecology surgery, infusion of 1000 ml of Hartmanns solution led to reduced PONV (Elhakim *et al.* 1998). In a similar study, fluids reduced late nausea but not vomiting (Spencer 1988). Giving a similar group 150 ml of clear fluid p.o. 2 hours before surgery did not alter rates of PONV (Goodwin *et al.* 1991). A double-blind trial of 20 ml/kg of fluid vs 2 ml/kg pre-operatively in ambulatory surgery patients showed less nausea at 24 hours in the group given additional fluids, but no difference in early nausea or vomiting (Yogendran *et al.* 1995).

Post-operative pain

Post-operative pain increases the incidences of PONV after abdominal surgery; the administration of opioids to relieve pain alleviated the nausea in 80% of cases (Andersen & Krohg 1976). It would appear that this area has not been revisited since this paper and its relevance to current practice is unclear.

Post-operative fluids

The effects of timing of post-operative administration of oral fluids on PONV are unclear. Schreiner and Woods have suggested a reduction of up to 50% in PONV before discharge from hospital when oral fluids were withheld from children after adeno-tonsillectomy and strabismus surgery. One group was randomised to mandatory fluids and the other given fluid on request, but this strategy did not reduce the overall incidence of PONV over 24 hours, as many children vomited during the journey home or at home (Schreiner *et al.* 1992). When a similar study was done in adult ambulatory patients there was no difference in PONV between those given a mandatory drink and those where fluids were withheld (Jin *et al.* 1998).Van den Berg reported that in adults and children who had undergone ophthalmic surgery, withholding oral fluids for at least 4 hours did not affect the overall incidence of PONV. However, in this study, half of those who vomited did so with their first oral fluid intake (van den Berg *et al.* 1987). These studies suggest that oral fluids after surgery should be lead by the wishes of the patient.

Predicting PONV

In an initial study Palazzo used logistic regression using five factors to develop a model predicting PONV in patients undergoing minor orthopaedic surgery (Palazzo & Evans 1993). The model was subsequently validated in patients undergoing other surgery (Toner *et al.* 1996). Further models have been constructed including those by Koivuranta *et al.* (1997), Sinclair *et al.* (1999) and Apfel *et al.* (1999).

Apfel further determined the risks of vomiting for four factors: female gender, history of motion sickness or PONV, non-smoking and post-operative opioids. The incidences of PONV were 10%, 21%, 39%, 61% and 79% with the presence of none, one, two three or four factors. The paper suggested that prophylactic therapy be instigated if two or more factors were present (Apfel *et al.* 1999).

The scoring systems mentioned above and two others were compared by Apfel (Apfel *et al.* 2002). None had a better than 70% chance of predicting PONV and those models using the most factors were no better at predicting PONV than simpler ones.

The apparent inability of scoring systems to predict the incidence of PONV with greater then 70% accuracy may be due to several factors (Apfel *et al.* 2002). The coupling of risk factors may explain the apparent lack of additional predictive power of those scoring systems with multiple variables. The models may not consider factors such as starvation, fluid and oxygen therapy, and movement, which may be hard to standardise between institutions. The considerable variation between and within individuals may also prevent any model being significantly more accurate.

Conclusion

What should we do with this information? Patient and surgical factors are beyond the control of the anaesthetist. However, we can choose our anaesthetic technique. Risk of PONV is probably minimised by using a technique with propofol and an opioid or a regional technique while avoiding nitrous oxide. Adequate fluid replacement and oxygenation are also sensible and risk free. Should we use intravenous anaesthesia for every case? Many clinicians are daunted by the apparent complexity and cost of intravenous anaesthesia and worry about perioperative awareness. Although these concerns may be ill founded they must be respected. Should patients have high levels of inspired oxygen even if their haemoglobin saturation is adequate at a lower level? If prediction of PONV were a precise art i.e. both sensitive and specific, then we could target our efforts at those patients at greatest risk. It is not enough to predict the risk in a population of patients because clinicians treat patients individually, and if predictions are to be useful they must work at an individual level as well. When the Palazzo scoring system was tested prospectively in 400 patients it was reasonably predictive of population risk, predicting an incidence of PONV of 36%, when the actual incidence was 27.4% (Palazzo & Evans 1993). However, when multiple models for predicting PONV were tested by Apfel none was correct more than 70% of the time and those with more factors to their model were no more accurate than simpler models (Apfel *et al.* 2002). Therefore, predictions for individuals are imperfect and those patients not identified as at risk may be denied techniques which could have minimised their morbidity. As we cannot predict risk for individuals we can consider treating populations. The appropriateness of this strategy must balance the cost and risk of treating prophylactically that subset of the patient population who are in fact at low risk/no risk. At present, we cannot reliably identify these individuals to whom treatment offers cost and risk but little or no benefit.

We are further hindered by the minimal data comparing different strategies. Does the addition of one or more prophylactic anti-emetics to an inhalational technique give a lower risk of PONV than an intravenous technique? Does the use of anti-emetics make an IV technique 'even better' or would they simply add risk of drug-related side effects without reducing morbidity? At present we do not know.

The patient, procedural and pharmacological factors associated with PONV have now been clearly defined and a framework for PONV studies established. Future work is needed to define the interaction of these factors and the cost-effectiveness of different strategies for reducing or preventing PONV.

References

Andersen, R. & Krohg, K. (1976). Pain as a major cause of postoperative nausea. *Canadian Anesthesiologists Society Journal* **23**(4), 366–369.

Aouad, M.T., Siddik, S.S., Rizk, L.B., Zaytoun, G.M., Baraka, A.S. (2001). The effect of dexamethasone on postoperative vomiting after tonsillectomy. *Anesthesia and Analgesia* **92**(3), 636–640.

Apfel, C.C., Kranke, P., Eberhart, L., Roos, A., Roewer, N. (2002). Comparison of predictive models for postoperative nausea and vomiting. *British Journal of Anaesthesia* **88**(2), 234–240.

Apfel, C.C., Läärä, E., Koivuranta, M., Greim, C-A., Roewer, N. (1999). A Simplified Risk Score for Predicting Postoperative Nausea and Vomiting Conclusions from Cross-validations between Two Centers. *Anesthesiology* **91**, 693–700.

Bacic, A., Rumboldt, Z., Gluncic, I., Buklijas, J. (1998). The impact of the menstrual cycle and ondansetron on postoperative nausea and vomiting. *International Journal of Clinical Pharmacology Research* **18**(4),153–158.

Beattie, W.S., Lindblad, T., Buckley, D.N., Forrest, J.B. (1991). The incidence of postoperative nausea and vomiting in women undergoing laparoscopy is influenced by the day of menstrual cycle. *Canadian Journal of Anesthesia* **38**(3), 298–302.

Bellville, J.W. (1961). Postanesthetic nausea and vomiting. *Anesthesiology* **22**, 773–780.

Bellville, J.W., Bross, I.D.J., Howlans, W.S. (1960). Post operative nausea and vomiting. IV. Factors related to post operative nausea and vomiting. *Anesthesiology* **6**, 186–193.

Bonica, J., Crepps, W., Monk, M., Bennett, B. (1958). Postanaesthetic nausea, retching and vomiting. *Anesthesiology* **19**, 532–540.

Bree, S.E., West, M.J., Talylor, P.A., Kestin, I.G. (1998). Combining propofol with morphine in patient-controlled analgesia to prevent postoperative nausea and vomiting. *British Journal of Anaesthesia* **80**(2), 152–154.

Carpenter, R.L., Caplan, R.A., Brown, D.L., Stephenson, C., Wu, R. (1992). Incidence and risk factors for side effects of spinal anesthesia. *Anesthesiology* **76**(6), 906–916.

Chalmers, I., Altman, D.G., editors. *Systematic reviews*. London: BMJ Publishing Group, 1995.

Chimbira, W., Sweeney, B.P. (2000). The effect of smoking on postoperative nausea and vomiting. *Anaesthesia* **55**(6), 540–544.

Chung, F., Mezei, G. (1999). Factors contributing to a prolonged stay after ambulatory surgery. *Anesthesia and Analgesia* **89**(6), 1352–1359.

Chung, F., Mezei, G., Tong, D. (1999). Adverse events in ambulatory surgery. A comparison between elderly and younger patients. *Canadian Journal of Anesthesia* **46**(4), 309–321.

Clarke, R.S. (1984). Nausea and vomiting. *British Journal of Anaesthesia* **56**(1), 19–27.

Cohen, M.M., Cameron, C.B., Duncan, P.G. (1990). Pediatric anesthesia morbidity and mortality in the perioperative period. *Anesthesia and Analgesia* **70**(2), 160–167.

Cook, R.J., Sackett, D.L. (1995). The number needed to treat: a clinically useful measure of treatment effect [published erratum appears in BMJ 1995 Apr 22;310(6986):1056]. *British Medical Journal* **310**(6977), 452–454.

Coveney, E., Weltz, C.R., Greengrass, R., Inglehart, J.D., Leight, G.S., Steele, S.M., Lyerly, H.K. (1998). Use of paraverebral block anesthesia in the surgical management of breast cancer. Experience in 156 cases. *Annals of Surgery* **227**(4), 496–501.

D'Alessio, J.G., Rosenblum, M., Shea, K.P., Freitas, D.G. (1995). A retrospective comparison of interscalene block and general anaesthesia for ambulatory shoulder arthroscopy surgery. *Regional Anesthesia* **20**(1), 62–68.

Datta, S., Alper, M.H., Ostheimer, G.W., Weiss, J.B. (1982). Method of ephedrine administration and nausea and hypotension during spinal anesthesia for cesarean section. *Anesthesiology* **56**(1), 68–70.

Dent, S., Ramachandra, V., Stephen, C.R. (1955). Postoperative vomiting: incidence, analysis and therapeutic measures in 3,000 patients. *Anesthesiology* **16**, 564–572.

Elhakim, M., el-Sebiae, S., Kaschef, N., Essawi, G. (1998). Intravenous fluid and postoperative nausea and vomiting after day-case termination of pregnancy. *Acta Anaesthesiologica Scandinavica* **42**(2), 216–219.

Flagg, P.J. *The Art of Anaesthesia*. 1st ed. Philadelphia: Lippincott, 1916.

Gan, T., Sloan, F., Dear Gde, L., El-Moalem, H.E., Lubarsky, D.A. (2001). How much are patients willing to pay to avoid postoperative nausea and vomiting? *Anesthesia and Analgesia* **92**(2), 393–400.

Gold, M.I. (1969). Postanesthetic vomiting in the recovery room. *British Journal of Anaesthesia* **41**(2), 143–149.

Goll, V., Akca, O., Greif, R., Freitag, H., Arkilic, C., Scheck, T., Zoeggeler, A., Kurz, A., Krieger, G., *et al.* (2001). Ondansetron is no more effective than supplemental intraoperative oxygen for prevention of postoperative nausea and vomiting. *Anesthesia and Analgesia* **92**(1), 112–117.

Goodwin, A., Rowe, W., Ogg, T., Samaan, A. (1991). Oral fluids prior to day surgery. The effect of shortening the pre-operative fluid fast on postoperative morbidity. *Anaesthesia* **46**(12),1066–8.

Greif, R., Laciny, S., Rapf, B., Hickle, R.S., Sessler, D.I. (1999). Supplemental oxygen reduces the incidence of postoperative nausea and vomiting. *Anesthesiology* **91**, 1246–1252.

Handa, F., Fujii, Y. (2001). The efficacy of oral clonidine premedication in the prevention of postoperative vomiting in children following strabismus surgery. *Paediatric Anaesthesia* **11**(1), 71–74.

Harmon, D., O'Connor, P., Gleasa, O., Gardiner, J. (2000). Menstrual cycle irregularity and the incidence of nausea and vomiting after laparoscopy. *Anaesthesia* **55**(12), 1164–1167.

Holt, R., Rask, P., Coulthard, K.P., Sinclair, M., Roberts, G., Van der Walt, J.H., MacKenzie, V., Rasmussen, M. (2000). Tropisetron plus dexamethasone is more effective than tropisetron alone for the prevention of postoperative nausea and vomiting in children undergoing tonsillectomy. *Paediatric Anaesthesia* **10**(2), 181–188.

Honkavaara, P., Lehtinen, A.M., Hovorka, J., Korttila, K. (1991). Nausea and vomiting after gynaecological laparoscopy depends upon the phase of the menstrual cycle. *Canadian Journal of Anesthesia* **38**(7), 876–879.

Honkavaara, P., Pyykko, I., Rutanen, E.M. (1996). Increased incidence of retching and vomiting during periovulatory phase after middle ear surgery. *Canadian Journal of Anesthesia* **43**, 1108–1114.

Hovorka, J., Korttila, K., Erkola, O. (1989). Nitrous oxide does not increase nausea and vomiting following gynaecological laparoscopy. *Canadian Journal of Anesthesia* **36**(2), 145–148.

Hovorka, J., Korttila, K., Erkola, O. (1990). The experience of the person ventilating the lungs does influence postoperative nausea and vomiting. *Acta Anaesthesiologica Scandinavica* **34**(3), 203–205.

Hovorka, J., Korttila, K., Erkola, O. (1990). Gastric aspiration at the end of anaesthesia does not decrease postoperative nausea and vomiting. *Anaesthesia and Intensive Care* **18**(1), 58–61.

Hovorka, J., Korttila, K., Nelskyla, K., Soikkeli, A., Sarvela, J., Paatero, H., Halonen, P., Yli-Hankala, A. (1997). Reversal of neuromuscular blockade with neostigmine has no effect on the incidence or severity of postoperative nausea and vomiting. *Anesthesia and Analgesia* **85**(6), 1359–1361.

Jenkins, K., Grady, D., Wong, J., Correa, R., Armanious, S., Chung, F. (2001). Post-operative recovery: day surgery patients' preferences. *British Journal of Anaesthesia* **86**(2), 272–274.

Jin, F., Norris, A., Chung, F., Ganeshram, T. (1998). Should adult patients drink fluids before discharge from ambulatory surgery? *Anesthesia and Analgesia* **87**(2), 306–311.

Jobalia, N., Mathieu, A. (1994). A meta-analysis of published studies confirms decreased postoperative nausea/vomiting with propofol. *Anesthesiology* **81**(3A), A33.

Kamath, B., Curran, J., Hawkey, C., Beattie, A., Gorbutt, N., Guiblin, H., Kong, A. (1990). Anaesthesia, movement and emesis. *British Journal of Anaesthesia* **64**(6), 728–730.

Kim, S.I., Han, T.H., Kil, H.Y., Lee, J.S., Kim, S.C. (2000). Prevention of postoperative nausea and vomiting by continuous infusion of subhypnoitc propofol in female patients receiving intravenous patient controlled analgesia. *British Journal of Anaesthesia* **85**(6), 898–900.

King, M.J., Milazkiewicz, R., Carli, F., Deacock, A.R. (1988). Influence of neostigmine on postoperative vomiting. *British Journal of Anaesthesia* **61**(4), 403–406.

Kober, A., Fleischackl, R., Scheck, T., Lieba, F., Strasser, H., Friedmann, A., Sessler, D.I. (2002). A Randomized Controlled Trial of Oxygen for Reducing Nausea and Vomiting During Emergency Transport of Patients Older Than 60 Years With Minor Trauma. *Mayo Clinic Proceedings* **77**(1), 35–38.

Koivuranta, M., Laara, E., Snare, L., Alahuhta, S. (1997). A survey of postoperative nausea and vomiting. *Anaesthesia* **52**(5), 443–449.

Konvalinka, P.A. (1999). Relationship of the menstrual cycle to postoperative incidence of emesis after laparoscopic cholecystectomy. *Clin Excell Nurse Pract* **3**(6), 353–358.

Kranke, P., Apfel, C.C., Papenfuss, T., Rauch, S., Loebmann, U., Ruebsam, B., Griem, C-A., Roewer, N. (2001). An increased body mass index is no risk factor for postoperative nausea and vomiting. *Acta Anaesthesiologica Scandinavica* **45**(2), 160–166.

Lerman, J., Eustis, S., Smith, D.R. (1986). Effect of droperidol pretreatment on postanesthetic vomiting in children undergoing strabismus surgery. *Anesthesiology* **65**(3), 322–325.

Lin, D.M., Furst, S.R., Rodarte, A. (1992). A double-blinded comparison of metoclopramide and droperidol for prevention of emesis following strabismus surgery. *Anesthesiology* **76**(3), 357–361.

Linbland, T., Forrest, J.B., Buckley, D.N., Beattie, W.S. (1990). Anaesthesia decreases a hormone mediated threshold for nausea and vomiting. *Anesthesia and Analgesia* **70**, S242.

Macario, A., Weinger, M., Carney, S., Kim, A. (1999). Which clinical anesthesia outcomes are important to avoid? The perspective of patients. *Anesthesia and Analgesia* **89**(3), 652–658.

McLeskey, C.H., Walawander, C.A., Nahrwold, M.L., Roizen, M.F., Stanley, T.H., Thisted, R.A., White, P.F., Apfelbaum, J.L., Grasela, T.H., *et al.* (1993). Adverse events in a multicenter phase IV study of propofol: evaluation by anesthesiologists and postanesthesia care unit nurses. *Anesthesia and Analgesia* **77**(4 Suppl), S3–S9.

Mikawa, K., Nishina, K., Maekawa, N., Obara, H.. (1995). Oral clonidine premedication reduces vomiting in children after strabismus surgery. *Canadian Journal of Anesthesia* **42**(11), 977–981.

Mirakhur, R.K. (1991). Anticholinergic drugs in anaesthesia. *Br J Hosp Med* **46**(6), 409–411.

Mojica, J.L., Melendez, H.J., Bautista, L.E. (2002). The Timing of Intravenous Crystalloid Administration and Incidence of Cardiovascular Side Effects During Spinal Anesthesia: The Results from a Randomized Controlled Trial. *Anesthesia and Analgesia* **94**(2), 432–437.

Montgomery, J.E., Sutherland, C.J., Kestin, I.G., Sneyd, J.R. (1996). Infusions of subhypnotic doses of propofol for the prevention of postoperative nausea and vomiting. *Anaesthesia* **51**(6), 554–557.

Muir, J.J., Warner, M.A., Offord, K.P., Buck, C.F., Harper, J.V., Kunkel, S.E. (1987). Role of nitrous oxide and other factors in postoperative nausea and vomiting: a randomized and blinded prospective study. *Anesthesiology* **66**(4), 513–518.

Mukherjee, K., Esuvaranathan, V., Streets, C., Johnson, A., Carr, A.S. (2001). Adenotonsillectomy in children: a comparison of morphine and fentanyl for peri-operative analgesia. *Anaesthesia* **56**(12), 1193–1197.

Myles, P., Williams, D., Hendrata, M., Anderson, H., Weeks, A. (2000). Patient satisfaction after anaesthesia and surgery: results of a prospective survey of 10,811 patients. *British Journal of Anaesthesia* **84**(1), 6–10.

Nelskyla, K., Yli-Hankala, A., Soikkeli, A., Korttila, K. (1998). Neostigmine with glycopyrrolate does not increase the incidence or severity of postoperative nausea and vomiting in outpatients undergoing gynaecological laparoscopy. *British Journal of Anaesthesia* **81**, 757–760.

Nelskyla, K.A., Yli-Hankala, A.M., Puro, P.H., Korttila, K.T. (2001). Sevoflurane titration using bispectral index decreases postoperative vomiting in phase II recovery after ambulatory surgery. *Anesthesia and Analgesia* **93**(5), 1165–1169.

Palazzo, M., Evans, R. (1993). Logistic regression analysis of fixed patient factors for postoperative sickness: a model for risk assessment. *British Journal of Anaesthesia* **70**(2), 135–140.

Palazzo, M.G., Strunin, L. (1984). Anaesthesia and emesis. I: Etiology. *Canadian Anesthesiologists Society Journal* **31**(2), 178–187.

Pataky, A., Kitz, D., Andrews, R., Lecky, J. (1988). Nausea and vomiting following ambulatory surgery: Are all procedures created equal? *Anesthesia and Analgesia* **67**, S163.

Purkis, I. (1964). Factors that influence postoperative vomiting. *Canadian Journal of Anaesthesia* **11**, 335–353.

Puttick, N., Van der Walt, J.H. (1987). The effect of premedication on the incidence of postoperative vomiting in children after E.N.T. surgery. *Anaesthesia and Intensive Care* **15**(2), 158–162.

Ratra, C.K., Badola, R.P., Bhargava, K.P. (1972). A study of factors concerned in emesis during spinal anaesthesia. *British Journal of Anaesthesia* **44**(11), 1208–1211.

Rowley, M.P., Brown, T.C. (1982). Postoperative vomiting in children. *Anaesthesia and Intensive Care* **10**(4), 309–313.

Rubin, A., Metz-Rubin, H. (1951). Effect of dramamine upon postoperative nausea and vomiting. *Surgery, Gynecology And Obstetrics* **92**, 415–418.

Salmenpera, M., Kuoppamaki, R., Salmenpera, A. (1992). Do anticholinergic agents affect the occurrence of postanaesthetic nausea? *Acta Anaesthesiologica Scandinavica* **36**(5), 445–448.

Schlager, A., Mitterschiffthaler, G., Puhringer, F. (2000). Rectally administered dimenhydrinate reduces postoperative vomiting in children after strabismus surgery. *British Journal of Anaesthesia* **84**(3), 405–406.

Schreiner, M.S., Nicolson, S.C., Martin, T., Whitney, L. (1992). Should children drink before discharge from day surgery? *Anesthesiology* **76**(4), 528–533.

Sinclair, D., Chung, F., Mezei, G. (1999). Can postoperative nausea and vomiting be predicted? *Anesthesiology* **91**(1), 109–118.

Smith, B.L., Manford, M.L. (1974). Postoperative vomiting after paediatric adenotonsillectomy. A survey of incidence following differing pre- and postoperative drugs. *British Journal of Anaesthesia* **46**(5), 373–378.

Sneyd, J.R., Carr, A., Byrom, W.D., Bilski, A.J. (1998). A meta-analysis of nausea and vomiting following maintenance of anaesthesia with propofol or inhalational agents. *European Journal of Anaesthesiology* **15**(4), 433–445.

Snow, J. (1991). *On Narcotism by the Inhalation of vapours, 1848*: Facsimile Edition. Royal Society of Medicine Services Ltd, London., 1848.

Spencer, E. (1988). Intravenous fluids in minor gynaecological surgery. Their effect on postoperative morbidity. *Anaesthesia 1988 Dec;43(12):1050-1* **43**(12), 1050–1051.

Splinter, W.M. (2001). Prevention of vomiting after strabismus surgery in children: dexamethasone alone versus dexamethasone plus low-dose ondansetron. *Paediatric Anaesthesia* **11**(5), 591–595.

Splinter, W.M., Rhine, E.J. (1998). Low-dose ondansetron with dexamethasone more effectively decreases vomiting after strabismus surgery in children than does high-dose ondansetron. *Anesthesiology* **88**(1), 72–75.

Swann, D.G., Spens, H., Edwards, S.A., Chestnut, R.J. (1993). Anaesthesia for gynaecological laparoscopy – a comparison between the laryngeal mask airway and tracheal intubation. *Anaesthesia* **48**(5), 431–434.

Toner, C.C., Broomhead, C.J., Littlejohn, I.H., Samra, G.S., Powney, J.G., Palazzo, M.G., Evans, S.J., Strunin, L. (1996). Prediction of postoperative nausea and vomiting using a logistic regression model. *British Journal of Anaesthesia* **76**(3), 347–351.

Tramer, M., Moore, A., McQuay, H. (1997a). Meta-analytic comparison of prophylactic antiemetic efficacy for postoperative nausea and vomiting: propofol anaesthesia vs omitting nitrous oxide vs total i.v. anaesthesia with propofol. *British Journal of Anaesthesia* **78**(3), 256–259.

Tramer, M., Moore, A., McQuay, H. (1997b). Propofol anaesthesia and postoperative nausea and vomiting: quantitative systematic review of randomized controlled studies. *British Journal of Anaesthesia* **78**(3), 247–255.

Trepanier, C.A., Isabel, L. (1993). Perioperative gastric aspiration increases postoperative nausea and vomiting in outpatients. *Canadian Journal of Anesthesia* **40**(4), 325–328.

van den Berg, A.A., Lambourne, A., Clyburn, P.A. (1989). The oculo-emetic reflex. A rationalisation of postophthalmic anaesthesia vomiting. *Anaesthesia* **44**(2), 110–117.

van den Berg, A.A., Lambourne, A., Yazji, N.S., Laghari, N.A. (1987). Vomiting after ophthalmic surgery. Effects of intra-operative antiemetics and postoperative oral fluid restriction. *Anaesthesia* **42**(3), 270–276.

Vance, J.P., Neill, R.S., Norris, W. (1973). The incidence and aetiology of post-operative nausea and vomiting in a plastic surgical unit. *British Journal of Plastic Surgery* **26**(4), 336–339.

Wang, S.M., Kain, Z.N. (2000). Preoperative anxiety and postoperative nausea and vomiting in children: is there an association? *Anesthesia and Analgesia* **90**(3), 571–575.

Warner, L.O., Rogers, G.L., Martino, J.D., Bremer, D.L., Beach, T.P. (1988). Intravenous lidocaine reduces the incidence of vomiting in children after surgery to correct strabismus. *Anesthesiology* **68**(4), 618–621.

Watcha, M.F., White, P.F. (1992). Postoperative nausea and vomiting. Its etiology, treatment, and prevention. *Anesthesiology* **77**(1), 162–184.

Yogendran, S., Asokumar, B., Cheng, D.C., Chung, F. (1995). A prospective randomized double-blinded study of the effect of intravenous fluid therapy on adverse outcomes on outpatient surgery. *Anesthesia and Analgesia* **80**(4), 682–686.

PART 2

Evidence and opinion for clinical intervention

Chapter 3

Non-pharmacological interventions in post-operative nausea and vomiting (PONV): the role of alternative and complementary therapies in prevention and management

Karen H. Simpson

Introduction

Post-operative nausea and vomiting (PONV) is a still major problem and many suggestions have been made for rationalising its management (Tramer 2001a, b). This review concentrates on the evidence for, and role of, acupuncture techniques for the prevention and treatment of PONV. References to the use of acupuncture began to appear in the English medical literature about 150 years ago (Saks 1991). Interest declined over the early part of the 20th century and has re-emerged in the past 30 years. A survey in 1995 assessed 8745 people and found that 1 in 4 used complementary medicine; acupuncture was used by 12% of those people. Acupuncture is popular again in the UK, illustrated by two recent studies of adverse events during acupuncture that surveyed about 66,000 acupuncture treatments during a relatively short timescale (MacPherson *et al.* 2001; White *et al.* 2001). The use of acupuncture is widespread in the USA where a National Institutes of Health Consensus Conference (1998) estimated that more than one million Americans have acupuncture treatment each year.

Evaluation of complementary therapies

Complementary therapies need to be evaluated carefully. The test of time is insufficient evidence upon which to base therapies. Rigorous assessment of efficacy is as important for acupuncture, as for any mainstream treatment. Acupuncture should only be integrated into routine care if it is proved to be effective after proper evaluation. Over the past ten years there have been several large systematic reviews of acupuncture published. A Cochrane field devoted to complementary medicine has been established (Ezzo *et al.* 1998). There are four well-supported indications for acupuncture using the available evidence: dental pain, low back pain, migraine and emesis (Ernst 1999; Mayer 2000). There are many indications where many randomised controlled trials have been published, but systematic reviews are inconclusive e.g. addiction, headache and neck pain. The evidence for acupuncture efficacy for treatment of smoking and obesity is conclusively negative.

ust be protected from useless treatments. Purchasers of health care have igation to use resources for the greatest good. They need accurate and nates of the cost benefits of complementary techniques as well as evidence fficacy and safety. Effective, safe and cheap therapies should be identified so that they can be integrated into conventional medicine. Inclusion of acupuncture into mainstream clinical care depends not only on its efficacy, but also on factors such as ease of use, cost and safety. The use of acupuncture requires training and competency assessment of therapists. There are no reliable cost comparisons of acupuncture compared with more conventional treatments. Acupuncture is not risk free, but life-threatening complications are rare (MacPherson *et al.* 2001; White *et al.* 2001).

Acupuncture research

Researchers need to be aware that clinical trials of acupuncture need a different set of methodological assumptions than drug trials. However, research design in acupuncture trials still needs to meet all conventional methodological requirements. There are obstacles to rigorous acupuncture research and studies of acupuncture often score quite low for methodological quality (National Institutes for Health Consensus Conference on Acupuncture 1998). There is a need for more good quality research (Mayer 2000). There are some unique difficulties when trying to design good acupuncture trials:

- There are many different forms of acupuncture treatment – it is not just one simple therapy. Acupuncture with needles, injection, acupressure, laser or electrical stimulation on the whole body or sometimes in confined areas such as the ear or hand are all used. These treatments may not be directly comparable and so interpretation of studies can be difficult.
- The diagnosis used to plan treatment is not always traditional. Each patient is treated as fairly unique. Chinese diagnoses that do not seem scientifically valid are sometimes used to make treatment plans.
- Therapy is often not standardised. Each patient may be treated differently and individuals may have different treatments on different occasion depending on the clinical response to each treatment.
- Children are often strong responders to acupuncture.
- Acupuncture by formula is not ideal and is different to the traditional method of treatment. Failure to demonstrate efficacy of acupuncture performed using a standard recipe for all patients is not equivalent to showing ineffectiveness of traditional acupuncture.
- The skill of the therapist may vary depending on their training and experience.
- Acupuncture points are of varying size and depth. They can also vary within the individual depending on whether they are healthy or not. There are many schools of thought about acupuncture points. However most acupuncturists are in agreement

that it necessary to produce 'needling sensation' or 'de qi' during treatment. It is probable that patients need to be conscious during acupuncture stimulation for it to be effective.

- Acupuncture can sometimes worsen the condition it is being used to treat. This is called 'aggravation'. It is commoner on those who are sensitive to acupuncture.
- Blinding during acupuncture trials is difficult. Patients in non-acupuncture groups must believe that they are having an effective treatment. Blinding of the operator is not possible; an independent person must do all the observations.
- The use of suitable control groups is difficult. It is possible that in some individuals, who are very sensitive to acupuncture, any point can produce an effect if stimulated. Any peripheral stimulation can modulate sensory input to the central nervous system. Noxious peripheral stimulation can mediate analgesia. Therefore any stimulus that pierces the skin cannot be regarded as a control. Therefore the needling of so called 'sham' points may not be the same as no treatment at all. A suitable placebo must be indistinguishable from the real intervention in all respects, e.g. appearance and sensation. There have been interesting developments with sham needles that may provide partial solutions to some of these problems.
- The use of a placebo treatment is one of the most difficult issues in acupuncture research. Acupuncture has all the attributes of a powerful placebo. When using electrical acupuncture it may be easier to provide a placebo by using subthreshold stimulation or not passing electrical current in the placebo group.
- Enthusiasts often do research. This may lead to biases, for example, they may be reluctant to publish negative results.

Considering all the difficulties with acupuncture research it would appear that studying the use of the technique in the treatment of PONV might be valuable. Many of the difficulties with acupuncture trials can be reduced when studying emesis. Nausea and vomiting can often be simpler to treat with acupuncture than many other conditions. It may be managed in some cases using a single point that is often the same for different individuals; this is the P6 point on the ventral wrist surface. There is a short follow up time when dealing with PONV. There is a reproducible end point with objective outcome measures. However, the mechanisms for nausea and vomiting differ, therefore the effect of acupuncture may be different for these two modalities.

Acupuncture for PONV

A systematic review examined acupuncture trials for the management of emesis performed before March 1995 (Vickers 1996). Forty-two trials were found on the use of P6 stimulation for PONV, cancer therapy or pregnancy related emesis. Papers were ranked after assessment of their methodological robustness. Nine papers were excluded after assessment (all of which favoured acupuncture). The method of P6 stimulation varied: manual or electrical (11), manual acupressure (4), wristbands (2), TENS (2) and injection (2). The use of controls varied: - none (9), historical (1), acupuncture under general anaesthesia (5), acupuncture with local anaesthesia (1), dummy points (1), placebo wrist bands (2) and sham TENS (2). Four trials of P6 acupuncture under general anaesthesia showed no effect. Twenty-seven of the remaining 29 studies showed an effect with acupuncture. There were only 12 randomised, placebo controlled trials of P6 acupuncture not under general anaesthesia; 11 of the 12 showed an effect for acupuncture. Eight of the randomised placebo controlled trials concerned PONV:

- P6 acupuncture vs dummy acupuncture vs no treatment control, $n = 75$ females, minor gynaecological surgery, number of patients symptom free after surgery = acupuncture 76%, dummy acupuncture 24%, control 24% ($p < 0.001$) (Dundee *et al.* 1986).
- P6 acupuncture vs no treatment control, $n = 500$ males and females, general surgery, incidence of vomiting = acupuncture 4.4% controls 16% ($p < 0.001$) (Fry 1986).
- Wristbands vs dummy wristbands vs prochlorperazine, $n = 152$ males and females, general surgery, nausea days 1 and 2 = wrist bands less than dummy bands and prochlorperazine ($p < 0.02$), nausea days 3–6 = no difference (Barsoum *et al.* 1990).
- P6 acupuncture after injection of local anaesthetic vs P6 acupuncture after injection of saline, $n = 74$ females, minor gynaecological surgery, symptom free within 6 hours of surgery = local anaesthesia 52%, saline 81% ($p < 0.013$) (Dundee & Ghaly1991).
- Wristband vs dummy wristbands, $n = 66$ children, squint surgery, number vomiting within 24 hours = wristbands 92%, controls 83%, not significant (Lewis *et al.* 1991).
- P6 acupressure vs dummy acupressure vs no treatment, $n = 90$ females, minor gynaecological surgery = P6 acupressure better than dummy acupressure or no treatment for nausea within first 6 hours after surgery (Gieron *et al.* 1993).
- P6 TENS stimulation vs sham TENS at P6, $n = 103$ females after hysterectomy = TENS better than sham TENS for control of vomiting during 36 hours after surgery (Fassoulaki *et al.* 1993).
- P6 TENS full stimulation vs P6 TENS subthreshold stimulation vs P6 sham TENS vs no treatment, $n = 230$ male and females, orthopaedic surgery = TENS full stimulation reduced sickness severity in females only ($p < 0.001$) (McMillan 1994).

The review showed that seven different centres had used different ways to stimulate P6 in adults and children of different sexes. A further study in 1994 that involved 46 women having gynaecological surgery was not included in the review (Allen *et al.* 1994). Those who had P6 stimulation rather than sham treatment had no difference in PONV, but had a reduced requirement for anti-emetic.

A literature search from March 1995 to 2002 revealed 17 more trials on the use of acupuncture stimulation for PONV. Five studies were excluded either because of methodological problems or in one case because the study was designed to look at post-operative pain and any change in emesis was incidental to the study. Therefore 12 further studies merit consideration. Among these are four studies that used different acupuncture techniques, for example stimulation of points other than P6, hand acupuncture and indwelling intradermal needles.

- P6 wrist bands vs placebo, $n = 60$, females post-Caesarean section under regional block with spinal opioid, emesis reduced for 48 hours with P6 wristbands (Ho *et al.* 1996).
- Transcutaneous stimulation of P6 and LI4 vs no treatment administered after anaesthesia, $n = 84$ children, no significant difference between groups (Schwager *et al.* 1996).
- P6 wrist bands vs dummy wrist bands, $n = 200$ males and females, short surgery, incidence of emesis = P6 group 23% and dummy group 41% ($p < 0.0058$) (Fan *et al.* 1997).
- P6 stimulation after anaesthesia but before opioid treatment vs no stimulation, $n = 81$ females, minor gynaecological day case surgery, P6 group decreased PONV for 24 hours after surgery. Acupuncture helped a subset of patients with a prior history of PONV and motion sickness. Placebo group had 16 times risk of PONV while in hospital and 4 times risk in 24 hours after discharge, 3 of placebo group had to be admitted to hospital because of emesis (Al-Sadi *et al.* 1997).
- P6 wristbands vs metoclopramide vs placebo, $n = 75$ females after Caesarean section, P6 wristbands and metoclopramide reduced emesis compared with placebo (Stein *et al.* 1997).
- P6 stimulation by laser vs placebo, $n = 40$ children after strabismus surgery, vomiting within 24 hours = P6 25%, placebo 85% ($p < 0.0001$) (Schlager *et al.* 1998).
- P6 acupressure vs placebo, $n = 104$ females undergoing laparoscopy, PONV within 24 hours = P6 acupressure 19% placebo 42% ($p < 0.005$) (Harmon *et al.* 1999)
- P6 acupressure vs placebo stimulation vs no treatment, $n = 60$ females undergoing day case gynaecological surgery = vomiting and need for rescue anti-emetic reduced by P6 acupressure ($p < 0.05$) (Alkaissi *et al.* 1999).
- BL10, BL11 and GB34 (acupuncture points pressured pre-operatively and needle-less plasters post-operatively vs placebo, $n = 65$ children undergoing strabismus surgery = early and late vomiting reduced by acupuncture ($p < 0.05$) (Chu *et al.* 1998).

- Pre-operative acupressure and intra/post-operative acupuncture of P6 vs sham treatment of P6, $n = 100$ children undergoing tonsillectomy = no significant effect on PONV (Shenkman *et al.* 1999).
- Korean hand acupressure vs placebo acupressure, $n = 80$ children undergoing strabismus surgery = vomiting reduced by acupuncture 20% vs placebo 68% ($p < 0.01$) (Schlager *et al.* 2000).
- Pre-operative insertion of indwelling intradermal needles in UB acupuncture points vs placebo, $n = 175$ males and females undergoing upper and lower abdominal surgery = acupuncture decreased PONV in upper abdominal surgery 24% vs placebo 50% ($p < 0.05$), acupuncture decreased PONV in lower abdominal surgery 18% vs placebo 47% ($p < 0.01$). Pain, opioid use and the humeral response to surgery were also reduced by acupuncture (Kotani *et al.* 2001).
- Transcutaneous electrical stimulation of P6 needles vs sham needles at P6 vs placebo, $n = 221$ males and females undergoing day case laparascopic cholecystectomy = nausea was decreased by active treatment ($p < 0.01$), vomiting was unaffected (Zarate *et al.* 2001).
- Electrical stimulation at P6 vs sham needle stimulation vs placebo, $n = 120$ children undergoing tonsillectomy = nausea reduced by active P6 treatment 60% vs sham 88% vs placebo 93% ($p < 0.01$). Vomiting and the use of rescue medication not affected (Rusy *et al.* 2002).

Conclusions

Overall, the evidence for acupuncture efficacy in the treatment of PONV in adults is good. However, much of the work has been done in adult females; only 24% of adult subjects in the 22 randomised controlled trials were male (Table 3.1). It is not clear if the findings in women are transferable to males. There has been little work done in children – only 22% patients in the 22 RCTs. There have been seven randomised studies of children using acupuncture while the subjects were conscious. Three that

Table 3.1 Acupuncture in the treatment of PONV

Numbers of patients included in all 30 studies of acupuncture for PONV

Total patients $n = 3060$		
Adults $n = 2404$	Males	451 (19%)
	Females	1953 (81%)
Children $n = 656$	(21%)	

Numbers of patients included in 22 randomised controlled trials of acupuncture for PONV

Total patients $n = 2505$		
Adults $n = 1950$	Males	462 (24%)
	Females	1488 (76%)
Children $n = 555$	(22%)	

stimulated P6 with pressure or TENS showed no effect. One that used laser and one that used electrical needling of P6 showed anti-emetic effects. Two that used other points and hand acupuncture reduced vomiting.

Acupuncture may be useful in the management of PONV. It may be a useful alternative or adjunct to multi-modal anti-emetic therapy. However, a scientific approach to complementary techniques is vital if they are to be integrated into clinical practice.

References

Allen, D.L., Kitching, A. J. & Nagle, C. (1994). P6 acupressure and nausea and vomiting after gynaecological surgery. *Anaesthesia and Intensive Care* **22**, 691–693.

Alkaissi, A. *et al.* (1999). Effect and placebo effect of acupressure (P6) on nausea and vomiting after outpatient gynaecological surgery. *Acta Anaesthesiologica Scandinavica* **43**, 270–274.

Al-Sadi, M., Newman, B. & Julious, S.A. (1997). Acupuncture in the prevention of post-operative nausea and vomiting. *Anaesthesia* **52**, 658–661.

Barsoum, G., Perry, E.P. & Fraser, I.A. (1990). Postoperative vomiting is relieved by acupressure. *Journal of the Royal Society of Medicine* **83**, 86–89.

Chu, Y.C., Lin, S.M., Hsieh, Y.C. *et al.* (1998). Effect of BL-10 (tianzhu), BL-11 (dazhu) and GB-34 (yanglinquan) acuplaster for prevention of vomiting after strabismus surgery in children. *Acta Anaesthesiologica Singapore* **36**, 11–16.

Dundee, J.W., Chestnutt, W.N., Ghaly, R.G. *et al.* (1986). Traditional Chinese acupuncture: a potentially useful antiemetic? *British Medical Journal* **293**, 583–584.

Dundee, J.W. & Ghaly, R.G. (1989). Does the timing of P6 acupuncture influence its efficacy as a postoperative antiemetic? *British Journal of Anaesthesia* **63**, 630P.

Dundee, J.W. & Ghaly, R.G. (1991). Local anaesthesia blocks the antiemetic action of P6. *Clinical Pharmacology and Therapeutics* **50**, 78–80.

Dundee, J.W. & Young, J. (1990). Prophylactic antiemetic action of acupuncture in patients having cancer chemotherapy. *Journal of the Royal Society of Medicine* **83**, 360–362.

Ernst, E. (1999). The clinical effectiveness of acupuncture: an overview of systematic reviews. In *Acupuncture, a Scientific Appraisal* (ed. Ernst, E. & White, A.), pp. 107–127. Butterworth Heinemann, Oxford.

Ezzo, J., Berman, B.M. & Vickers, A.J. *et al.* (1998). Complementary medicine and the Cochrane collaboration. *Journal of the American Medical Association* **280**, 1628–1630.

Fan, C.F., Tanhiu, E., Joshi, S. *et al.* (1997). Acupressure treatment for prevention of postoperative nausea and vomiting. *Anesthesia and Analgesia* **84**, 821–825.

Fassoulaki, A., Papils, K., Sarantopoulos, C. *et al.* (1993). Transcutaneous electrical nerve stimulation educes the incidence of vomiting after hysterectomy. *Anaesthesia and Analgesia* **76**, 1012–1014.

Fry, E.N.S. (1986). Acupressure and postoperative vomiting. *Anaesthesia* **41**, 661–662.

Gieron, C., Wieland, B., von der Laage, D. *et al.* (1993). Acupressure in the prevention of postoperative nausea and vomiting. *Anaesthetist* **42**, 221–226.

Harmon, D. *et al.* (1999). Acupressure and the prevention of nausea and vomiting after laparoscopy. *British Journal of Anaesthesia* **82**, 387–390.

Ho, C.M., Hseu, S.S., Tsai, S.K. *et al.* (1996). Effect of P6 acupressure on prevention of nausea and vomiting after epidural morphine for post-cesarean section pain relief. *Acta Anaesthesiologica Scandinavica* **40**, 372–375.

Kotani, N., Hashimoto, H., Sato, Y. *et al.* (2001). Preoperative intradermal acupuncture reduces postoperative pain, nausea and vomiting, analgesic requirement, and sympathoadrenal responses. *Anesthesiology* **95**, 349–356.

Lee, A. & Done, M.L. (1999). The use of non-pharmacological techniques to prevent PONV: a meta-analysis. *Anesthesia and Analgesia* **88**, 1362–1369.

Lewis, I.H., Pryn, S.J., Reynolds, P.I. *et al.* (1991). Effect of P6 acupressure on postoperative vomiting in children undergoing outpatient strabismus correction. *British Journal of Anaesthesia* **67**, 73–78.

MacPherson, H., Thomas, K., Walters, S. *et al.* (2001). The York acupuncture safety study: prospective survey of 34 000 treatments by traditional acupuncturists. *British Medical Journal* **323**, 486–487.

Mayer, D.J. (2000). Acupuncture: an evidence-based review of the clinical literature. *Annual Reviews in Medicine* **51**, 49–63.

McMillan, C.M. (1994). Transcutaneous electrical stimulation of Neiguan antiemetic acupuncture point in controlling sickness following opioids analgesia in major orthopaedic surgery. *Physiotherapy* **80**, 5–9.

National Institutes for Health Consensus Conference on Acupuncture (1998). *Journal of the American Medical Association* **280**, 1518–1524.

Rusy, L.M., Hoffman, G.M. & Weisman, S.J. (2002). Electroacupuncture prophylaxis of postoperative nausea and vomiting following pediatric tonsillectomy with or without adenoidectomy. *Anesthesiology* **96**, 300–305.

Saks, M. (1991). The flight from science? The reporting of acupuncture in British mainstream journals from 1800 to 1990. *Complementary Medicine Research* **5**, 178–183.

Schlager, A., Offer, T. & Baldissera, I. (1998). Laser stimulation of acupuncture point P6 reduces postoperative vomiting in children undergoing strabismus surgery. *British Journal of Anaesthesia* **81**, 529–533.

Schlager, A., Boehler, M. & Puhringer, F. (2000). Korean hand acupressure reduces postoperative vomiting in children after strabismus surgery. *British Journal of Anaesthesia* **85**, 267–270.

Schwager, K.L., Baines, D.B. & Meyer, R.J. (1996). Acupuncture and postoperative vomiting in day-stay paediatric patients. *Anaesthesia and Intensive Care* **24**, 674–677.

Shenkman, Z., Holzman, R.S., Kim, C. *et al.* (1999). Acupressure–acupuncture antiemetic prophylaxis in children undergoing tonsillectomy. *Anesthesiology* **90**, 1311–1316.

Stein, D.J., Birnbach, D.J., Danzer, B.I. *et al.* (1997). Acupressure versus intravenous metoclopramide to prevent nausea and vomiting during spinal anaesthesia for cesarean section. *Anesthesia and Analgesia* **84**, 342–345.

Tramer, M.R. (2001a). A rational approach to the control of postoperative nausea and vomiting: evidence from systematic reviews. Part 1. Efficacy and harm of antiemetic interventions, and methodological issues. *Acta Anaesthesiologica Scandinavica* **45**, 4–14.

Tramer, M.R. (2001b). A rational approach to the control of postoperative nausea and vomiting: evidence from systematic reviews. Part II. Recommendations for prevention and treatment, and research agenda. *Acta Anaesthesiologica Scandinavica* **45**, 14–20.

Vickers, A.J. (1996). Can acupuncture have specific effects on health? A systematic review of acupuncture anti-emesis trials. *Journal of the Royal Society of Medicine* **89**, 303–311.

White, A., Hayhoe, S., Hart, A. *et al.* (2001). Adverse events following acupuncture: prospective survey of 32 000 consultations with doctors and physiotherapists. *British Medical Journal* **323**, 485–486.

Zarate, E., Mingus, M., White, P.F. *et al.* (2001). The use of transcutaneous acupoint electrical stimulation for postoperative nausea after laparascopic surgery. *Anesthesia and Analgesia* **92**, 629–635.

Chapter 4

Pharmacological intervention in post-operative nausea and vomiting: scientific evidence and expert opinion for anti-emetic therapy for prophylaxis and management

Michael Harmer

Background to therapy

The basis for the pharmacological control of post-operative nausea and vomiting (PONV) centres around the mechanisms and receptors involved in the sensory, processing and motor actions involved in its production. The mechanisms involved in this process are ever-evolving as we gain a better understanding of the interrelationships between physical, chemical and emotional sensory inputs that result in the processes of vomiting and, perhaps even more unpleasant, nausea. It has equally become apparent that the mechanisms cannot be the same for the two modalities and they are not of necessity linked, with nausea possible without vomiting or retching (an unproductive vomiting act), and vice versa.

Sensory Inputs

For the specific area of PONV, it is probably acceptable to use a simple scheme of receptor interaction to explain why certain drugs may lead to PONV whereas others may reduce or eliminate it. The main afferent inputs that may stimulate PONV are shown in Figure 4.1.

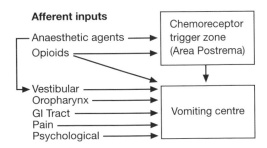

Figure 4.1 Physiology of PONV.

Although the vomiting centre has little anatomical meaning, it is a physiological concept that has been accepted as a representation of the central processing unit for vomiting (though possibly not for nausea). Further details of the physiology of PONV can be found in Andrews' excellent review which forms Chapter One of the current volume.

The main afferent inputs are: opioids, anaesthetic agents, pain, vestibular and oropharyngeal stimulation, gastrointestinal receptors, and psychological. Many of these inputs are influenced by anaesthesia or the peri-operative period:

Opioids and pain

Opioids are potent stimulators of nausea and vomiting, and a common component of most general anaesthetics. They are also widely used in the post-operative period to treat pain. Avoidance may be helpful but an alternative analgesic regimen must be employed as pain itself is a potent stimulator of nausea and vomiting. The move in recent years towards an increased use of regional technique, for post-operative pain management has lead to some improvements.

Anaesthetic agents

Many of the older agents such as ether and methohexitone were well recognised as potent stimulators of PONV. However, even currently used agents such as etomidate are known to cause PONV and, unless specifically indicated on other grounds, might sensibly be avoided in routine practice. In addition, nitrous oxide has been incriminated to some extent, with the mechanism probably relating to increases in air space volume subsequent upon it replacing nitrogen; thus there may be gut distension or increased middle ear pressure. Finally, the use of neostigmine to reverse the effects of neuromuscular block has been linked to PONV. Modern neuromuscular blocking agents are often used in infusions and allowed to 'wear off' rather than needing reversal.

Vestibular and oropharyngeal stimulation

In addition to any effect of nitrous oxide on the middle ear, anaesthesia almost certainly sensitises the vestibular apparatus. The handling of patients in the immediate post-operative period with sudden changes of position and direction of movement is very likely to cause vestibular stimulation and subsequent PONV. Equally, the persistent use of pharyngeal suctioning, often with a rigid sucker, can have a profound stimulating effect on the vomiting process.

Gastrointestinal inputs

It seems self evident that a patient with a full stomach is more likely to suffer PONV than a starved patient. However, it may not be quite that simple as it would seem that small quantities of clear fluid, rather than being detrimental may be advantageous in promoting gastric emptying and hence reducing the incidence (or volume) of vomiting.

Psychological

The peri-operative patient undergoes a wide range of psychological experiences including fear, anxiety, depression, elation, relief, pain, etc. Allaying of any, or all, of these may help considerably in reducing the incidence of PONV. In the patient where clear explanation and discussion does not work, there may be a place for an anxiolytic.

Thus careful, thoughtful peri-operative care can do much to reduce the necessity for prevention or treatment strategies.

Receptors involved in PONV

The pharmacology that has evolved for the management of PONV has centred largely upon the receptors thought to be involved. Much of the evidence upon which these receptors have been identified has come from animal models or from extrapolation from other areas of clinical practice in which nausea and vomiting are common problems. This may lead to some inconsistencies as there is not a good animal model for vomiting and the afferent inputs involved in such areas as chemotherapy may be very different to those in PONV. However, it has 'traditionally' been accepted that several receptors were involved in nausea and vomiting (Table 4.1).

Table 4.1 Receptors traditionally accepted as involved in the process of PONV

Receptor type	Site of action
Dopamine	Chemoreceptor trigger zone
Opioid	(Area Postrema)
$5\text{-}HT_3$	
Cholinergic	Vomiting centre
Histamine	
Opioid	
? Neurokinin$_1$	

NB: Refer to Andrews (Chapter One) for a detailed exposition of current receptor physiology

Drugs used in the prevention and treatment of PONV

Drug therapy is based upon the receptor types believed to be involved in PONV and so is basically divided into: anti-dopaminergic, anti-histaminic, anti-cholinergic and anti-serotonergic drugs. In addition, there are a group of miscellaneous drugs such as steroids, ginger and cannabinoids that appear to have an anti-emetic effect but without a clear receptor-based mechanism.

Anti-dopaminergic drugs

These drugs exhibit a range of activity at the dopaminergic receptor as well as having other effects. For example, metoclopramide has prokinetic effects, droperidol has sedative and autonomic effects whereas prochlorperazine has hypnotic properties. As a group, they have been used for PONV for many years.

Metoclopramide is a substituted benzamide first developed in the early 1960s. Its main action as an anti-dopaminergic is on the chemoreceptor trigger zone and it has prokinetic effects in enhancing gastric and upper intestinal motility. Metoclopramide also has some weak serotonin receptor activity (in particular 5-HT$_3$).

In his review of the management of PONV, Rowbotham (1992) showed a wide range of efficacy for metoclopramide, with several studies where metoclopramide was not considered statistically to be any better than placebo.

Scrutiny of the more recent, randomised, controlled studies of metoclopramide in PONV have shown a very similar picture (Table 4.2). The wide variability in patient type, operation type, definition of PONV and design of studies, makes comparison between different studies largely meaningless.

Table 4.2 Summary of recent studies on metoclopramide.

Reference	Type of Patient	Type of Surgery	Type of Study (Comparators)	Incidence of PONV
Lacroix (1996)	Adults	General surgery	Prevention R,DB (droperidol, propofol)	24%
Watts (1996)	Adults	Day case laparoscopic	Prevention R (ondansetron, cyclizine)	24%
Wilson (2001)	Adults	Outpatient laparoscopic cholecystectomy	Prevention R,DB,PC** (ondansetron)	32%
Woodward (1999)	Adults	Cardiac surgery	Prevention R,DB (ondansetron)	34%
Diemunsch (1997a)	Adults	General	Treatment R,DB (ondansetron)	59%
Fujii (1998a)	Adult females with previous PONV	Major gynaecological	Prevention R,DB (droperidol, granisetron)	60%
Nagiub (1996)	Adults	Laparoscopic cholecystectomy	Prevention R,DB,PC* (droperidol, tropisetron, granisetron)	71%
Scuderi (1997)	Child	Outpatient strabismus	Prevention R,DB,PC* (droperidol, ondansetron)	32%

R, randomised; DB, double blind; PC, placebo controlled; *, no difference to placebo; **, significant difference to placebo.

The incidence of vomiting ranges from 24% to 71% in a variety of studies involving different types of surgery, patients and hospital setting (inpatient vs. outpatient). As such, it is very difficult to differentiate one aspect from another. However, it is interesting to note that in one of the placebo-controlled studies shown in Table 4.2, metoclopramide showed no significant difference to placebo. Thus, one is left with a very similar impression to that of Rowbotham (1992) that metoclopramide in adults has a limited role as an anti-emetic in the peri-operative period, though it may have a place on account of its prokinetic effects.

There have been very few studies in children with the only placebo-controlled study by Scuderi *et al.* (1997) showing an incidence of vomiting of 32% which was not statistically different from placebo.

A meta-analysis by Domino *et al.* (1999) showed metoclopramide to be less effective than ondansetron or droperidol. Another meta-analysis by Henzi *et al.* (1999) showed it to have little action on nausea but some effect on vomiting.

Side effects

The most important side effects of metoclopramide are extrapyramidal reactions. These are more common in young female patients with a proposed incidence of 1 in 5000 in the 12–19 year age range (Bateman *et al.* 1965). Sedation occurs in approximately 10% of patients receiving long-term therapy (Harrington *et al.* 1983) but is seldom a problem when used for the treatment of PONV. Some authors have reported restlessness, agitation and akathisia after normal doses of metoclopramide (Dundee & Clarke 1973; Caldwell *et al.* 1987).

Metoclopramide has also been associated with significant decreases of blood pressure (Pegg 1980) and increase in heart rate (Ellis & Spence 1970). It is thus recommended that intravenous metoclopramide should be given over 1–2 minutes.

The overall impression of metoclopramide in clinical practice is shown in Table 4.3.

Table 4.3 Overall impression of metoclopramide

Benefits	Drawbacks
Widely used in clinical practice	Limited efficacy (?any better than placebo)
Useful prokinetic effects	Not as effective as ondansetron or droperidol
Possibility of an intranasal preparation	Extrapyramidal side effects
	Possible problems with gastrointestinal surgery

Alizapride has only been studied once but was found to be effective (Stienstra *et al.* 1997) being comparable to droperidol and ondansetron.

Droperidol is a butyrophenone and within the same family as major psychotrophic drugs such as haloperidol. Droperidol is a known potent neuroleptic and was developed for use in such a role. However, used in small doses, less than 5 mg (and often as little as 0.25 mg), it has been shown to have anti-emetic properties.

A review of recent randomised, controlled studies in which droperidol has been used is presented in Table 4.4.

Table 4.4 Summary of recent studies on droperidol

Reference	Type of Patient	Type of Surgery	Type of Study (Comparators)	Incidence of PONV
Lacroix (1996)	Adults	General surgery	Treatment R,DB (propofol, metoclopramide)	4%
Maestre (1997)	Adults	Ambulatory	Prevention R,DB,PC* (metoclopramide, ondansetron)	6%
Gan (1994)	Adults	Hip and knee replacement	Prevention R,DB,PC** (ondansetron)	18%
Loo (1997)	Adult females	Minor gynaecology	Prevention R (droperidol + metoclopramide)	23%
Fabling (2000)	Adults	Craniotomy	Prevention R, DB, PC** (ondansetron)***	25%
Peixoto (2000)	Adults	Major gynaecology	Prevention R, DB (ondansetron/both) ***	33%
Wang (1999)	Adult females	Thyroidectomy	Prevention R, DB, PC ** (dexamethasone) ***	35%
Bugedo (1999)	Adults	Biliary, gynaecology	Prevention R, DB, PC ** (ondansetron) ***	37%
Reihner (2000)	Adult females	Breast	Prevention R, DB, PC ** (ondansetron) ***	48%
Janknegt (1999)	Adult females	Gynaecology, breast and ENT	Prevention R, DB (granisetron, granisetron and dexamethasone) +	52%
Scuderi (1997)	Children	Outpatient strabismus	Prevention R,DB,PC** (metoclopramide, ondansetron)	5%
Shende (2001)	Children	Strabismus	Prevention R, DB, PC ** (ondansetron) ***	32%
Goodarzi (1998)	Children (2-14 years)	Major orthopaedic	Prevention R,DB,PC** (ondansetron)	40%

R, randomised; DB, double blind; PC, placebo controlled; *, no difference to placebo; **, significant difference to placebo; ***, no difference to comparator; +, comparator superior.

The incidence of vomiting in these adult studies shows a huge range, from 4% to 52% for a wide variety of operations and other variables. Several studies were placebo controlled and in most, droperidol was statistically better than the placebo.

There have been three recent placebo-controlled studies in children, with a huge difference in the incidence of vomiting (Scuderi *et al.* 1997; Shende *et al.* 2001; Goodarzi 1998). All three studies showed droperidol to be better than placebo.

In addition to its use as a prophylactic agent, droperidol has been used as an adjunct to patient-controlled analgesia. Walder & Aitkenhead (1995) found an overall PONV incidence of 40% in patients who had undergone major gynaecological surgery. However, the actual dose that is effective is open to debate as Lamond *et al.*

(1998) could find no difference in effect for a bolus dose range of 0.05–0.2 mg. In a comparator study of ondansetron versus droperidol used in a patient-controlled analgesia system, Millo *et al.* (2001) found no difference between the groups, though the incidence of PONV in both groups was high (49% droperidol, 61% ondansetron).

Side effects

The most common side effect is delay in recovery caused by sedation. This is more likely with larger doses but can occasionally occur even with lower doses. Extrapyramidal reactions are also a recognised problem. Anxiety (Thorpe & Smith 1996) and akathisia (Foster *et al.* 1996) have been reported after relatively small doses of droperidol. These problems seem to occur sometime after surgery and have lead to concerns over the use of droperidol for day-case surgery. Such concerns and commercial financial considerations have led to the withdrawal of droperidol from the UK market.

The overall impression of droperidol in clinical practice is shown in Table 4.5.

Table 4.5 Overall impression of droperidol

Benefits	Drawbacks
Widely used by anaesthetists (until withdrawn in UK)	Variable efficacy
	Many reports of side effects
Reasonable efficacy for prevention	
	Onset of side effects may be delayed
Considered a 'standard' for other drugs	
	Little evidence of 'treatment' effect
	Withdrawn from UK market

Haloperidol, although predominantly used as a major psychotrophic tranquiliser, has anti-emetic qualities (Judkins & Harmer 1982) when given orally as a premedicant.

Phenothiazines were originally developed in the late 19th century by chemists working in the dye industry. Later, promethazine was found to have profound hypnotic properties and from that compound the anti-emetic drugs, prochlorperazine and perphenazine have been developed.

In his review in 1992, Rowbotham observed that although prochlorperazine had been in clinical use since the 1950s for the prevention of PONV, there had been precious few studies. One recent study (Lee *et al.* 2000) has suggested that prochlorperazine is as effective as ondansetron 4 or 8 mg in the prevention of PONV after gynaecological laparoscopy; however, it should be stressed that none of the drugs seemed very effective in the particular clinical setting. In contrast, Chen *et al.* (1998) showed prochlorperazine to be more effective than ondansetron 4 mg in the prevention of PONV after total hip or knee replacement surgery. Although widely used in clinical practice in both prophylactic and treatment roles, it is only licensed for the latter indication and then only as a single dose.

To much the same extent, very little is known about perphenazine although favoured by many older anaesthetists as part of the 'recipe' for patients at high risk of PONV. However, the study by Steinbrook *et al.* (1998) showed perphenazine to be as effective as combinations of ondansetron plus droperidol, and metoclopramide plus droperidol.

Side effects

The major perceived side effect of phenothiazines is extrapyramidal reaction, though the evidence for such being any worse than other dopaminergic agents is scanty. However, one study (Robbie 1959) suggested that such reactions were more likely after perphenazine than prochlorperazine. As both drugs have sedative qualities, it is hardly surprising that they may cause delays in recovery from anaesthesia.

The overall impression of phenothiazines in clinical practice is shown in Table 4.6.

Table 4.6 Overall impression of phenothiazines

Benefits	Drawbacks
Widely used by ward staff	Variable efficacy
Perphenazine recently shown to be as effective as ondansetron	Many reports of side effects
	Very few controlled studies
Prochlorperazine may be comparable to ondansetron in some situations	Only licensed for treatment

Anti-cholinergics

The only anti-cholinergic that has been shown to have anti-emetic qualities is hyoscine. However, there have been very few studies on hyoscine used for PONV, with most of the literature dating back to before 1990. If administered intravenously, hyoscine can cause confusion and delayed recovery from anaesthesia. Although used primarily for its 'drying' effects, the traditional papaveretum/hyoscine ('om and scop') premedication may have had some anti-emetic benefits. Even so, dry mouth is a commom complaint of patients given hyoscine. In the management of motion sickness, transdermal hyoscine has been shown to be useful but when used for PONV, the patch has to be applied well in advance of the precipitary factors. It has been shown to be effective in the prevention of PONV after ear surgery (Honkavaara and Pyykko 1999).

Overall, there is a feeling, largely unsubstantiated by good clinical studies, that hyoscine may be a useful drug in patients where the chief stimulus to PONV is of a vestibular origin.

Anti-histaminics

Drugs of several types (e.g. piperazines, phenothiazines) exhibit histamine type-1 receptor antagonist activity and many are anti-emetics. Whereas many anti-histamines have been used in the management of motion sickness, only cyclizine has found a place in the treatment of PONV.

Cyclizine is a piperazine derivative and has anti-muscarinic in addition to anti-histaminic actions. The main body of studies of cyclizine date back to the 1960s and only a few have been done since then. However, cyclizine has grown in popularity for the treatment of PONV where anecdotally it seems to be as good as any other agent.

A study by Watts (1996) showed a rather disappointing incidence of PONV in day cases of 51% with cyclizine, which was comparable to that achieved in a pilot study when no anti-emetic therapy was given. A more recent study (Cholwill et al. 1999) in day-case gynaecological laparoscopy has shown cyclizine 50 mg to be as effective as ondansetron 4 mg in the prevention of PONV. Cyclizine has also been given in combination with patient-controlled analgesia morphine (Walder and Aitkenhead 1995). In this study, the incidence of PONV with cyclizine was 28%.

On the positive side, cyclizine seems to have few major side effects, in particular, there are no extrapyramidal side effects. Sedation and a dry mouth are often present; a consequence of the anti-muscarinic activity.

Cyclizine, for no real scientific reasons, does appear to have developed a niche in the treatment of PONV.

An anti-emetic effect is only associated with HT_1 receptor antagonists. A study with the H_2 receptor blocker, ranitidine, showed no difference to placebo (Cozanitis et al. 1996).

5-HT$_3$ antagonists

This group of drugs have evolved from the development of anti-emetics for use in chemotherapy-induced nausea and vomiting, particularly after cisplatin. The observation that high dose metoclopramide was partly effective in the prevention of cisplatin-induced nausea and vomiting lead to the discovery that the 5-HT$_3$ receptor was involved in the process. There can be little denying the dramatic effect that these drugs have had on chemotherapy-induced nausea and vomiting. However, the introduction of 5-HT$_3$ antagonists into practice for the prevention and treatment of PONV has not been so successful, possibly as a consequence of the limited involvement of 5-HT$_3$ release in the PONV process.

Ondansetron is probably the best investigated of the 5-HT$_3$ antagonists. Several studies have been undertaken on ondansetron, both compared with placebo and, more lately, active anti-emetics. A summary of recent randomised, controlled studies on ondansetron are shown in Table 4.7.

Table 4.7 Summary of recent studies on ondansetron

Reference	Type of Patient	Type of Surgery	Type of Study (Comparators)	Incidence of PONV
Maestre (1997)	Adults	Ambulatory	Prevention R,DB,PC * (metoclopramide, droperidol)	6%
Gan (1994)	Adults	Hip and knee replacement	Prevention R,DB,PC ** (droperidol)	17%
Tsui (1999)	Adult females	Gynaecological laparotomies	Prevention R, DB, PC ** (tropisetron) ***	18%
Watts (1996)	Adult females	Laparoscopic surgery	Prevention R, DB (cyclizine, metoclopramide)	20%
Goll (2001)	Adult females	Gynaecological laparoscopy	Prevention R (oxygen) ***	30%
Nagiub (1996)	Adults	Laparoscopic cholecystectomy	Prevention R, DB, PC ** (tropisetron, granisetron, metoclopramide)	34%
Sung (1993)	Adult females	Ambulatory gynaecology	Prevention R, DB, PC** (no active comparator)	38%
Diemunsch (1997a)	Adults	General surgery	Treatment R, DB (metoclopramide)	41%
Scuderi (1997)	Children	Outpatient strabismus	Prevention R, DB, PC** (metoclopramide, droperidol)	5%
Goodarzi (1998)	Children (2-14 years)	Major orthopaedic	Prevention R,DB,PC** (droperidol)	25%

R, randomised; DB, double blind; PC, placebo controlled; *, no difference to placebo;
, significant difference to placebo; *, comparator study, no difference.

In two paediatric studies (Scuderi *et al.* 1997; Goodarzi 1998), ondansetron was shown to be superior to placebo and, in the latter, to droperidol.

Granisetron has been investigated in several settings by predominantly one group. A summary of the studies is shown in Table 4.8.

In all studies containing a placebo control group there was a significant difference with granisetron.

Tropisetron has very similar properties and has conflictingly been shown to have less effect than ondansetron and granisetron (Naguib *et al.* 1996), and more effect than ondansetron (Pascucci *et al.* 1996).

Dolasetron has been available in the US since 1995 and in Germany since 1997 and more recently was launched in the UK. Comparative studies in a range of surgical settings have been conducted. Recent studies are summarised in Table 4.9.

Table 4.8 Summary of recent studies on granisetron

Reference	Type of Patient	Type of Surgery	Type of Study (Comparators)	Incidence of PONV
Fujii (1998d)	Adult females	Thyroid surgery	Prevention R,DB,PC**[with 100mcg/kg]* [with 20mcg/kg] (three doses of granisetron)	12% [100mcg/kg] 56% [20mcg/kg]
Fujii (1998c)	Adults	Middle ear surgery	Prevention R,DB (droperidol, metoclopramide)	15%
Fujii (1998b)	Adult females	Breast surgery	Prevention R,DB,PC** (droperidol, metoclopramide)	17%
Fujii (1998a)	Adult females with history of motion sickness	Major gynaecology	Prevention R,DB,PC** (droperidol, metoclopramide)	23%
Janknegt (1999)	Adult females	Gynaecology, breast and ENT	Prevention R, DB (droperidol) +	34%
Nagiub (1996)	Adults	Laparoscopic cholecystectomy	Prevention R,DB,PC** (tropisetron, ondansetron, metoclopramide)	48%

R, randomised; DB, double blind; PC, placebo controlled; *, no difference to placebo;
**, significant difference to placebo; +, superior to comparator.

Table 4.9 Summary of recent (1997) studies on dolasetron

Reference	Type of Patient	Type of Surgery	Type of Study (Comparators)	Incidence of PONV
Kortilla (1997)	Adults	Range of surgery	Prevention R,DB,PC** (ondansetron)	29% [50mg]
Diemunsch (1997)	Adult females	Gynaecology	Prevention R,DB,PC** (different doses of dolasetron)	33% [25mg]
Graczyk (1997)	Adult females	Laparoscopy	Prevention R,DB,PC** (different doses of dolasetron)	44% [50mg]
Warriner (1997)	Adult females	Abdominal hysterectomy	Prevention O,R,DB,PC** (different doses of dolasetron)	46% [100mg]
Diemunsch (1997)	Adults	Range of surgery	Treatment R,DB,PC** (different doses of dolasetron)	62% [50mg]
Kovac (1997)	Adults	Outpatient	Treatment R,DB,PC** (different doses of dolasetron)	65% [12.5mg]

See also Triem *et al.* (1999), Philip *et al.* (2000), Zarate *et al.* (2000), Danner *et al.* (2001), Piper *et al.* (2001), Walker (2001), Piper *et al.* (2002) & Burmeister *et al.* (2003)

O, oral; R, randomised; DB, double blind; PC, placebo controlled; *, no difference to placebo;
**, significant difference to placebo.

Other 'setrons' such as lerisetron and alosetron are currently under investigation for chemotherapy-induced nausea and vomiting, and may, in time, find their way into PONV practice.

Side effects

These are very rare with 5-HT$_3$ antagonists being restricted largely to headache. There is no evidence of extrapyramidal reactions. A recent comparative review of 5-HT$_3$ antagonists comments that small, statistically significant but clinically asymptomatic changes in electrocardiographic parameters have been reported. This appears to be a class effect with no significant difference in frequency among agents. Additionally, these electrocardiographic changes have not been associated with clinically significant cardiovascular sequelae (see Hesketh 2000). Overall, these drugs are considered to be well tolerated.

The overall impression of the 5-HT$_3$ drugs is shown in Table 4.10.

Table 4.10 Overall impression of 5-HT$_3$ receptor blockers

Benefits	Drawbacks
Shown to be highly effective in chemotherapy	? Effective against opioid-induced nausea and vomiting
Very low incidence of side effects	Expensive
Most effective of the currently available agents for both prevention and treatment	? Problems with QTc and arrhythmias
	Most effective when given in combination with other anti-emetics

Neurokinin 1 receptor antagonists

These are the latest generation of drugs undergoing investigation. They appear to act by preventing the vomiting process rather than by blocking the afferent input. In animal studies, these drugs appear able to prevent vomiting from any cause but whether they are effective in preventing nausea remains unclear. Early studies in humans showed promise that this effectiveness in animal work will be translated into humans; however, so far, such promise has not been realised.

Other treatments

Steroids have been shown to be effective in the prevention of PONV (Liu *et al.* 2001; Wang *et al.* 2000) and comparable to other agents (Wang *et al.* 1999). Dexamethasone has also been shown to have benefits in the extended post-operative period in children undergoing adenotonsillectomy (Pappas *et al.* 1998).

Propofol, given in low doses, has been said to reduce the incidence of PONV. However, recent studies by Lacroix *et al.* (1996) looking at the treatment of established PONV and by Montgomery *et al.* (1996) in the prevention of PONV have been unable to show an effect.

Cannabinoids have been suggested as effective anti-emetics. Most reports are anecdotal with the only comparison showing nabilone to be less effective than metoclopramide (Lewis *et al.* 1994).

Ginger is a well-recognised remedy used in motion and pregnancy-induced sickness. There is no convincing evidence of its superiority over placebo in the prevention of PONV.

PONV management options
Prevention

In considering the prevention options, the 5-HT$_3$ receptor antagonists appear to be the best option with the highest efficacy of the currently available drugs. This impression is further enhanced when the very limited side effect profile is taken into account. The addition of dexamethasone would seem to enhance the effectiveness.

Treatment

There have been very few studies looking at treatment. Cyclizine and prochlorperazine are widely used but the only comparative study shows a benefit of ondansetron over metoclopramide (Diemunsch *et al.* 1997) although dolasetron has been shown to be more effective than placebo. That coupled with the 'setrons' side effect profile suggests them to be reasonable drugs for this purpose.

To treat or to prevent?

There must remain a dilemma as to whether one should try to prevent PONV or treat it as and when it occurs. One factor that must be taken into account is the balance between efficacy of prevention and the incidence of side effects. If one uses a philosophy of the number-needed-to-treat to prevent one episode of PONV, one can have a measure of efficacy but often the incidence of side effects of the drugs is not so clear. In a study on PONV after squint surgery, Tramer *et al.* (1995) could show a definite efficacy/side effect ratio for ondansetron. Figures for other drugs or indications may not be so convincing.

References

Bateman, D.N., Rawlins, M.D. & Simpson, J.M. (1965). Extrapyramidal reactions to metoclopramide. *British Medical Journal* **291**, 930–932.

Bugedo, G., Gonzalez, J., Asenjo, C. *et al.* (1999). Ondansetron and droperidol in the prevention of postoperative nausea and vomiting. *British Journal of Anaesthesia* **83**, 813–814.

Burmeister, M.A., Standl, T.G., Wintruff, M., Brauer, P., Blanc, I. & Schulte am Esch, J. (2003). Dolasetron prophylaxis reduces nausea and postanaesthesia recovery time after remifentanil infusion during monitored anaesthesia care for extracorporeal shock wave lithotripsy. *British Journal of Anaesthesia* **90**, 194–198.

Caldwell, C., Rains, G. & McKiterick, K. (1987). An unusual reaction to preoperative metoclopramide. *Anesthesiology* **67**, 854–855.

Chen, J.J., Frame, D.G. & White, T.J. (1998). Efficacy of ondansetron and prochlorperazine for the prevention of postoperative nausea and vomiting after total hip replacement or total knee replacement procedures: a randomized, double-blind, comparative trial. *Archives of Internal Medicine* **158**, 2124–2128.

Cholwill, J.M., Wright, W., Hobbs, G.J. *et al.* (1999). Comparison of ondansetron and cyclizine for prevention of nausea and vomiting after day-case gynaecological laparoscopy. *British Journal of Anaesthesia* **83**, 611–614.

Cozanitis, D., Asantila, R., Eklund, P. *et al.* (1996). A comparison of ranitidine, droperidol or placebo in the prevention of nausea and vomiting after hysterectomy. *Canadian Journal of Anaesthesia* **43**, 106–109.

Danner, K., Becker, H.G., Best, B. & Madler, C. (2001). Prophylaxis of nausea and vomiting after thyroid surgery: comparison of oral and intravenous dolasetron with intravenous droperidol and placebo. *Anasthesiologie Intensivmedizin Notfallmedizin Schmerztherapie* **36**, 425–430.

Diemunsch, P., Conseiller, C., Clyti, N. *et al.* (1997a). Ondansetron compared with metoclopramide in the treatment of established postoperative nausea and vomiting. *British Journal of Anaesthesia* **79**, 322–326.

Diemunsch, P., D'Hollander, A., Paxton, L. *et al.* (1997b). Intravenous dolasetron mesilate in the prevention of postoperative nausea and vomiting in females undergoing gynecological surgery. *Journal of Clinical Anesthesia* **9**, 365–373.

Diemunsch, P., Leeser, J., Feiss, P. *et al.* (1997c). Intravenous dolasetron mesilate ameliorates postoperative nausea and vomiting. *Canadian Journal of Anaesthesia* **44**, 173–181.

Domino, K.B., Anderson, E.A., Polissar, N.L. *et al.* (1999). Comparative efficacy and safety of ondansetron, droperidol and metoclopramide for preventing postoperative nausea and vomiting, a meta-analysis. *Anesthesia and Analgesia* **88**, 1370–1399.

Dundee, J.W. & Clarke, R.S.J. (1973). The premedicant and anti-emetic action of metoclopramide. *Postgraduate Medical Journal* (Suppl.), 34–37.

Ellis, F.R. & Spence, A.A. (1970). Clinical trials of metoclopramide (Maxolon) as an antiemetic in anaesthesia. *Anaesthesia* **25**, 368–371.

Fabling, J.M., Gan, T.J., El-Moalem, H.E. *et al.* (2000). A randomized, double-blinded comparison of ondansetron, droperidol and placebo for prevention of postoperative nausea and vomiting after supratentorial craniotomy. *Anesthesia and Analgesia* **91**, 358–361.

Foster, P.N., Stickle, B.R. & Laurence, A.S. (1996). Akathisia following low-dose droperidol for antiemesis in day-case patients. *Anaesthesia* **51**, 491–494.

Fujii, Y., Saitoh, Y., Tanaka, H. *et al.* (1998a). Prevention of PONV with granisetron, droperidol or metoclopramide in patients with postoperative emesis. *Canadian Journal of Anaesthesia* **45**, 153–156.

Fujii, Y., Tanaka, H. & Toyooka, H. (1998b). Prevention of nausea and vomiting in female patients undergoing breast surgery: a comparison with granisetron, droperidol, metoclopramide and placebo. *Acta Anaesthesiologica Scandinavica* **42**, 220–224.

Fujii, Y., Toyooka, H. & Tanaka, H. (1998c). Prophylactic anti-emetic therapy with granisetron, droperidol and metoclopramide in female patients undergoing middle ear surgery. *Anaesthesia* **53**, 1165–1168.

Fujii, Y., Saitoh, Y., Tanaka, H. *et al.* (1998d). Prophylactic antiemetic therapy with granisetron in women undergoing thyroidectomy. *British Journal of Anaesthesia.* **81**, 526–528

Gan, T.J., Collis, R. & Hetreed, M. (1994). Double-blind comparison of ondansetron, droperidol and saline in the prevention of postoperative nausea and vomiting. *British Journal of Anaesthesia* **72**, 544–547.

Goll, V., Akca, O., Grief, R. *et al.* (2001). Ondansetron is no more effective than supplemental intraoperative oxygen for prevention of postoperative nausea and vomiting. *Anesthesia and Analgesia* **92**, 112–117.

Goodarzi, M. (1998). A double blind comparison of droperidol and ondansetron for prevention of emesis in children undergoing orthopaedic surgery. *Paediatric Anaesthesia* **8**, 325–329.

Graczyk, S.G., McKenzie, R., Kaller, S. *et al.* (1997). Intravenous dolasetron for the prevention of postoperative nausea and vomiting after outpatient laparoscopic gynecologic surgery. *Anesthesia and Analgesia* **84**, 325–330.

Harrington, R.A., Hamilton, C.W., Brogden. R.N. *et al.* (1983). Metoclopramide: an updated review of its pharmacological properties and clinical use. *Drugs* **25**, 451–494.

Henzi, I., Walder, B. & Tramer, M.R. (1999). Metoclopramide in the prevention of postoperative nausea and vomiting: a quantitative systematic review of randomised, placebo-controlled studies. *British Journal of Anaesthesia* **83**, 761–771.

Hesketh, P.J. (2000). Comparative review of 5-HT$_3$ receptor antagonists in the treatment of acute chemotherapy-induced nausea and vomiting. *Cancer Investigation* **18**, 163–173.

Honkavaara, P. & Pyykko, I. (1999). Effects of atropine and scopolamine on bradycardia and emetic symptoms in otoplasty. *Laryngoscope* **109**, 108–112.

Janknegt, R., Pinckaers, J.W., Rohof, M.H. *et al.* (1999). Double-blind comparative study of droperidol, granisetron and granisetron plus dexamethasone as prophylactic anti-emetic therapy in patients undergoing abdominal, gynaecological, breast or otolaryngological surgery. *Anaesthesia* **54**, 1059–1068.

Judkins, K.C. & Harmer, M. (1982). Haloperidol as an adjunct analgesic in the management of postoperative pain. *Anaesthesia* **37**, 1118–1120.

Kortilla, K., Clergue, F., Leeser, J. *et al.* (1997). Intravenous dolasetron and ondansetron in the prevention of postoperative nausea and vomiting: a multicenter, double-blind, placebo-controlled study. *Acta Anaesthesiologica Scandinavica* **41**, 914–922.

Kovac, A.L., Scideri, P.E., Boerner, T.F. *et al.* (1997). Treatment of postoperative nausea and vomiting with single intravenous doses of dolasetron mesylate: a multicenter trial. *Anesthesia and Analgesia* **85**, 546–552.

Lacroix, G., Lessard, M.R. & Trepanier, C.A. (1996). Treatment of post-operative nausea and vomiting: comparison of propofol, droperidol and metoclopramide. *Canadian Journal of Anaesthesia* **43**, 115–120.

Lamond, C.T., Robinson, D.L., Boyd, J.D. *et al.* (1998). Addition of droperidol to morphine administered by the patient-controlled analgesia method: what is the optimal dose? *European Journal of Anaesthesiology* **15**, 304–309.

Lee, T.H., Lin, C.G., Lee, T.C. *et al.* (2000). Failure of prevention against postoperative nausea and vomiting by ondansetron or prochlorperazine in patients undergoing gynaecological laparoscopy. *Acta Anaesthesiologica Sinica* **38**, 201–205.

Lewis, I.H., Campbell, D.N. & Barrowcliffe, M.P. (1994). Effect of nabilone on nausea and vomiting after total abdominal hysterectomy. *British Journal of Anaesthesia* **73**, 244–6.

Liu, Y.H., Li, M.J., Wang, P.C. *et al.* (2001). Use of dexamethasone on the prophylaxis of nausea and vomiting after tympanomastoid surgery. *Laryngoscope* **111**, 1271–1274.

Loo, C.C., Thomas, E., Tan, H.M. *et al.* (1997). A comparison of the antiemetic efficacy of droperidol alone and in combination with metoclopramide in day surgery anaesthesia *Medical Journal of Malaysia* **52**, 264–268.

Maestre, J.M., Puente, J. & Dierssen, T. (1997). Prevention of postoperative nausea and vomiting with metoclopramide, droperidol and ondansetron: a randomized, double-blind comparison with placebo in ambulatory surgery. *Ambulatory Surgery* **5**, 153–159.

Millo, J., Siddons, M., Innes, R. *et al.* (2001). Randomized, double-blind comparison of ondansetron and droperidol to prevent postoperative nausea and vomiting associated with patient-controlled analgesia. *Anaesthesia* **56**, 60–65.

Montgomery, J.E., Sutherland, C.J., Kestin, I.G. *et al.* (1996). Infusions of subhypnotic doses of propofol for the prevention of postoperative nausea and vomiting. *Anaesthesia* **51**, 554–557.

Nagiub, M., El Bakry, A.K., Kloshim, M.H.B. *et al.* (1996). Prophylactic antiemetic therapy with ondansetron, tropisetron, granisetron and metoclopramide in patients undergoing laparoscopic cholecystectomy: a randomized, double-blind comparison with placebo. *Canadian Journal of Anaesthesia* **43**, 226–231.

Pappas, A.L., Sukhani, R., Hotaling, A.J. *et al.* (1998). The effect of preoperative dexamethasone on the immediate and delayed postoperative morbidity in children undergoing adenotonsillectomy. *Anesthesia and Analgesia* **87**, 57–61.

Pascucci, G., Palmieri, V., Miranda, G. *et al.* (1996). Tropisetron versus ondansetron in the prevention and control of postoperative nausea and vomiting. *Acta Anaesthesiologica Italica* **47**, 173–177.

Peixoto, A.J., Peixoto Filho, A.J., Leaes, L.F. *et al.* (2000). Efficacy of prophylactic droperidol, ondansetron or both in the prevention of postoperative nausea and vomiting in major gynaecological surgery. A prospective, randomized, double-blind clinical trial. *European Journal of Anaesthesiology* **17**, 611–615.

Pegg, M.S. (1980). Hypotension following metoclopramide injection. *Anaesthesia* **35**, 614–616.

Philip, B.K., Pearman, M.H., Kovac, A.L. *et al.* (2000). Dolasetron for the prevention of post-operative nausea and vomiting following outpatient surgery with general anaesthesia: a randomised, placebo-controlled study. The Dolasetron PONV Prevention Study Group. *European Journal of Anaesthesiology* **17**, 23–32.

Piper, S.N., Triem, J.G., Maleck, W.H., Fent, M.T., Huttner, I. & Boldt, J. (2001). Placebo-controlled comparison of dolasetron and metoclopramide in preventing postoperative nausea and vomiting in patients undergoing hysterectomy. *European Journal of Anaesthesiology* **18**, 251–256.

Piper, S.N., Suttner, S.W., Rohm, K.D., Maleck, W.H., Larbig, E. & Boldt, J. (2002). Dolasetron, but not metoclopramide prevents nausea and vomiting in patients undergoing laparoscopic cholecystectomy. *Canadian Journal of Anaesthesia* **49**, 1021–1028.

Reinher, E., Grunditz, R., Giesecke, K. *et al.* (2000). Postoperative nausea and vomiting after breast surgery: efficacy of prophylactic ondansetron and droperidol in a randomized placebo-controlled study. *European Journal of Anaesthesiology* **17**, 197–203.

Robbie, D.S. (1959). Postanaesthetic vomiting and anti-emetic drugs. *Anaesthesia* **14**, 349–354.

Rowbotham, D.J. (1992). Current management of postoperative nausea and vomiting. *British Journal of Anaesthesia* **69** (Suppl. 1), 46S–59S.

Scuderi, P.E., Weaver, R.G. Jr, James, R.L. *et al.* (1997). A randomized double-blind, placebo controlled comparison of droperidol, ondansetron, and metoclopramide for the prevention of vomiting following outpatient strabismus surgery in children. *Journal of the Clinical Anesthesia* **9**, 551–558.

Shende, D., Bharti, N., Kathirval, S. *et al.* (2001). Combination of droperidol and ondansetron reduces PONV after paediatric strabismus surgery more than single drug therapy. *Acta Anaesthesiologica Scandinavica* **45**, 756–760.

Steinbrook, R.A., Gosnell, J.L. & Freiberger, D. (1998). Prophylactic antiemetics for laparoscopic cholecystectomy: a comparison of perphenazine, droperidol plus ondansetron, and droperidol plus metoclopramide. *Journal of Clinical Anesthesia* **10**, 494–498.

Stienstra, R., Samhan, Y.M., El-Mofty, M. *et al.* (1997). Double-blind comparison of alizapride, droperidol and ondansetron in the treatment of post-operative nausea. *European Journal of Anaesthesiology* **14**, 290–294.

Sung, Y.-F., Wetchler, B.V., Duncalf, D. *et al.* (1993). A double-blind, placebo controlled pilot study examining the effectiveness of intravenous ondansetron in the prevention of postoperative nausea and emesis. *Journal of Clinical Anesthesia* **5**, 22–29.

Thorpe, S.J. & Smith, A.F. (1996). A case of postoperative anxiety due to low dose droperidol used with patient-controlled analgesia. *International Journal of Obstetric Anesthesia* **5**, 283–284.

Tramer, M., Moore, A. & McQuay, H. (1995). Prevention of vomiting after paediatric strabismus surgery: a systematic review using the numbers-needed-to-treat method. *British Journal of Anaesthesia* **75**, 556–561.

Triem, J.G., Piper, S.N., Maleck, W.H., Schenck, A., Schmidt, C.C. & Boldt, J. (1999). Prevention of post-operative nausea and vomiting after hysterectomy with oral dolasetron, intravenous dehydrobenzperidol or a combination of both substances. *Anasthesiologie Intensivmedizin Notfallmedizin Schmerztherapie* **34**, 340–344.

Tsui, S.L., Ng, K.F., Wong, L.C. *et al.* (1999). Prevention of postoperative nausea and vomiting in gynaecological laparotomies: a comparison of tropisetron and ondansetron. *Anaesthesia and Intensive Care* **27**, 471–476.

Walder, A.D. & Aitkenhead, A.R. (1995). A comparison of droperidol and cyclizine in the prevention of postoperative nausea and vomiting associated with patient-controlled analgesia. *Anaesthesia* **50**, 654–656.

Walker, J.B. (2001). Efficacy of single dose intravenous dolasetron versus ondansetron in the prevention of postoperative nausea and vomiting. *Clinical Therapeutics* **23**, 932–938.

Wang, J.J., Ho, S.T., Lee, S.C. *et al.* (1999). The prophylactic effect of dexamethasone on postoperative nausea and vomiting in women undergoing thyroidectomy: a comparison of droperidol with saline. *Anesthesia and Analgesia* **89**, 200–203.

Wang, J.J., Ho, S.T., Lee, S.C. *et al.* (2000). The use of dexamethasone for preventing postoperative nausea and vomiting in females undergoing thyroidectomy: a dose-ranging study. *Anesthesia and Analgesia* **91**, 1404–1407.

Warriner, C.B., Knox, D., Belo, S. *et al.* (1997). Prophylactic oral dolasetron mesylate reduces nausea and vomiting after abdominal hysterectomy. *Canadian Journal of Anaesthesia* **44**, 1167–1173.

Watts, S.A. (1996). A randomized double-blinded comparison of metoclopramide, ondansetron and cyclizine in day-case laparoscopy. *Anaesthesia and Intensive Care* **24**, 546–551.

Wilson, E.B., Bass, C.S., Abramet, W. *et al.* (2001). Metoclopramide versus ondansetron in prophylaxis of nausea and vomiting for laparoscopic cholecystectomy. *American Journal of Surgery* **181**, 138–141.

Woodward, D.K., Sherry, K.M. & Harrison, D. (1999). Antiemetic prophylaxis in cardiac surgery: comparison of metoclopramide and ondansetron. *British Journal of Anaesthesia* **83**, 933–935.

Zarate, E., Watcha, M.F., White, P.F., Klein, K.W., Sa Rego, M. & Stewart, D.G. (2000). A comparison of the costs and efficacy of ondansetron versus dolasetron for anti-emetic prophylaxis. *Anesthesia and Analgesia* **90**, 1352–1358.

Chapter 5

Combination therapy and clinical decision making in situations of competing treatment options. What if anti-emetic therapy fails?

Imad T. Awad and David J. Rowbotham

Introduction

Post-operative nausea and vomiting (PONV) is regarded by many patients as the most unpleasant potential side effect after surgery and anaesthesia. Many anaesthetists are aware of this and will administer or prescribe an anti-emetic routinely. Despite this practice, many patients experience troublesome PONV. In this chapter, we shall explore factors that influence the failure of initial treatment and consider further therapeutic options. The use of combination therapy will also be reviewed.

There are two situations when failure of treatment becomes apparent. Firstly, in an individual patient complaining of PONV after anti-emetic therapy. Secondly, a high incidence of PONV may be detected in a population of patients, perhaps after clinical audit. Although many similar factors apply to both situations, we shall consider them separately.

Failure of treatment in an individual patient

There are various factors to be aware of when treatment in an individual patient has failed.

Has the drug been given?

In many cases, this may be the most important single factor in failure of treatment when an anti-emetic has been prescribed for post-operative use. There is evidence that anti-emetic therapy has a relatively low priority on the ward and that the utilisation of anti-emetic drugs by medical and nursing staff could be improved. This problem is discussed in detail in Chapter 8.

Has the drug been absorbed?

In most cases, anti-emetics are given intravenously or intramuscularly but they may be given orally, perhaps as premedication or on discharge to patients after day-case surgery. In this situation, oral bioavailability and rate of absorption may be an important factor in the failure of treatment.

Table 5.1 summarises the bioavailability and time to maximum plasma concentration (t_{max}) of some anti-emetics after oral administration. Data in the literature is often limited, particularly for the older anti-emetics (Rowbotham 1992). Metoclopramide is absorbed rapidly and the mean (range) t_{max} in volunteers was 0.9 (0.5–1.25) h (Ross-Lee et al. 1981). However, despite a bioavailability of 80%, there is enormous individual variation. For example, some subjects absorb only one third of the oral dose (Harrington et al. 1983). Prochlorperazine is poorly absorbed e.g. t_{max} range 1.5–5 h (Taylor et al. 1987), bioavailability 15% (Isah et al. 1992). Data for cyclizine are sparse. In one volunteer, t_{max} of 2 h was observed after administration of oral cyclizine 50 mg (Griffn & Baselt 1984). Ondansetron is quite well absorbed orally with a bioavailability of about 60% and t_{max} of 0.5–2 h (Roila & Delfavero 1995). Dolasetron is rapidly converted to its major metabolite (hydrodolasetron) which is active at the 5-HT$_3$ receptor (Balfour & Goa 1997). Median t_{max} of the metabolite after oral administration was approximately 1 h (Boxenbaum et al. 1993). These data are from patients or volunteers with normal gastric emptying.

Table 5.1 Oral absorption of some anti-emetics

Drug name	Bioavailability (%)	t_{max} (h)	Reference
Metoclopramide	80 (32–97)*	1–2.5	Harrington et al. (1983) Ross-Lee et al. (1981)
Prochlorperazine	15	2.8	Isah et al. (1992) Taylor & Bateman (1987)
Cyclizine		2	Griffn & Baselt (1984)
Ondansetron	60	0.5–2	Roila & Delfavero (1995)
Dolasetron	70	1**	Boxenbaum et al. (1993)
Granisetron	60	1.5–1.9	Kudoh et al. (1993)

*, Range; **, active metabolite.

In the perioperative period, many factors delay, or even inhibit completely, gastric emptying (Table 5.2). Opioid administration is particularly important in this context. Clearly, in the perioperative period, the absorption of any anti-emetic administered orally may be unreliable.

Has the appropriate dose been administered?

The drug may be ineffective because an inappropriate dose has been administered. With the exception of droperidol, only the recently introduced anti-emetic drugs have undergone extensive dose–response investigation. The recommended doses of cyclizine, prochlorperazine and metoclopramide have not been derived from appropriate dose ranging studies, primarily because they were introduced before strict licensing regulations. However, evidence suggests that the relative ineffectiveness of

Table 5.2 Important causes of delayed gastric emptying in the perioperative period

Causes of delayed gastric emptying	
Physiological	Pain
	Anxiety
Pathological	GI obstruction
	Acute gastritis
	Electrolyte imbalance
	Diabetes
Pharmacological	Opioids
	Anti-cholinergics
	Sympathomimetics

metoclopramide may be because the recommended dose (10 mg) is insufficient (Rowbotham 1992; Henzi et al. 1999). The dose–response relationship of droperidol has been investigated by in several clinical situations in an attempt to separate the anti-emetic effect from sedation (Rowbotham 1992).

Drugs introduced more recently such as ondansetron and dolasetron have undergone extensive investigation before licensing. Recommended doses are derived from specifically designed dose ranging studies. However, despite this, the correct dose may not be certain. For example, data from original studies on ondansetron suggested that a dose of 8 mg (rather than that of the recommended 4 mg) may be more appropriate for those with a previous history of PONV (McKenzie et al. 1993).

Is the drug still present?

The elimination half-lives of the commonly used anti-emetics vary widely (Table 5.3) and data are again sparse for the older drugs. Metoclopramide has a half-life of approximately 4 h (Harrington et al. 1983). The pharmacokinetics of prochlorperazine were published years after its introduction into clinical practice (Isah et al. 1992; Nahata et al. 1992; Taylor & Bateman 1987) and its half-life is longer than that of metoclopramide, although a study in children receiving chemotherapy revealed a large range (1.2–15.5 h). The limited data available indicates that cyclizine has a comparatively long half-life (Griffn & Baselt 1984; Walker & Kanfer 1996) compared with other anti-emetics.

The elimination half-life of droperidol is approximately 2 h (Cressman et al. 1973; Grunwald et al. 1993). The pharmacokinetics of the new 5-HT$_3$ antagonists are well described. For example, the elimination half-life of ondansetron is approximately 4 h (Roila & Delfavero 1995) and that of the active metabolite of dolasetron is 6.6–8.8 h (Dimmitt et al. 1999).

Despite the fact that anti-emetics are often ineffective, our knowledge of the pharmacokinetics of many anti-emetics is superficial. For example, there are few data available on the pharmacokinetics of infusion regimens and the time course of effector site concentrations. More work is required in this area.

Table 5.3 Half-lives of some anti-emetics

Name of drug	Half-life (h)	Reference
Metoclopramide	4	Harrington et al. (1983)
Prochlorperazine	6.8 7.5 5.6*	Taylor & Bateman (1987) Isah et al. (1992) Nahata et al. (1992)
Droperidol	2 1.7**	Cressman et al. (1973) Fischler et al. (1986) Grunwald et al. (1993)
Cyclizine	13	Walker & Kanfer (1996)
Ondansetron	3.8	Roila & Delfavero (1995)
Granisetron	2.9–6.3	Allen et al. (1994) Kudoh et al. (1993)
Dolasetron	6.6–8.8	Dimmitt et al. (1999)

*, Range 1.2–15.5 hours; **, children.

Is there a treatable cause for PONV?

One of the most important principles of medical practice is to treat the cause of a symptom before treating the symptom itself. There are many causes of PONV and several are treatable and potentially serious. It may be that the anti-emetic therapy has failed because a potent cause of PONV is present: all patients who do not respond to anti-emetic therapy should be assessed with this in mind.

Table 5.4 summarises the causes of PONV. Hypotension and hypoxaemia are common and important complications after anaesthesia and surgery. A frequent cause of PONV, particularly in the day-care setting, is forced fluid intake or mobilisation. If these are included as criteria for discharge, it may be that they are introduced at an inappropriately early stage in the patient's recovery. Forced fluid intake before discharge from the day ward was associated with increased incidence of PONV in children but not in adults (Marshall & Chung 1999). Psychological factors play an important role also and, if predominant, will often be associated with poor response to therapy. Occasionally, failure to respond to treatment may indicate abdominal or other pathology resulting from a surgical complication. This should be considered in all poor- or non-responders, particularly before discharge from the day-care unit.

Opioids are a common cause of PONV, especially if these drugs are being administered injudiciously. A more appropriate post-operative pain regimen such as regional analgesia and non-steroidal anti-inflammatory drugs may reduce the problem significantly. It should be remembered that other drugs can cause nausea and vomiting and, in the perioperative period, antibiotics are a common culprit. The use of these drugs should be reassessed if PONV is a severe problem.

What drug to use next?

Despite the factors discussed above, most patients in whom an anti-emetic has failed will require the administration of another anti-emetic. It is probably appropriate to choose a drug that acts by a different mechanism. This statement is not based on evidence from clinical trials in this situation because these data do not exist. However, there are some data about combination of anti-emetics for PONV prophylaxis (see below) and the strategy is consistent with the basic well-accepted pharmacological principles.

Table 5.5 summarises the potential sites of action of anti-emetics which have been reviewed in detail in Chapter One and the pharmacology of many of these drugs is discussed in Chapter Four. Metoclopramide, droperidol and prochlorperazine act primarily at the dopamine receptor and all are associated with extrapyramidal side effects. Cyclizine is predominantly anti-cholinergic. The 5-HT$_3$ antagonists such as ondansetron, dolasetron and granisetron are relatively effective and well tolerated and represent another group of drugs with a specific site of action. Antagonists at the NK$_1$ receptor are also anti-emetics and may be a useful therapeutic alternative in future (Fukuda *et al*. 1999; Gesztesi *et al*. 2000).

Table 5.4 Important causes of PONV

Hypotension
Hypoxaemia
Drugs – opioids
– antibiotics
Prolonged fasting pre-operatively
GI pathology
Psychological factors
Mobilisation
Fluid intake
NG tube
Pain

Table 5.5 Sites of action of anti-emetics

Antagonists

        Dopaminergic
        Cholinergic (M receptors)
        Histaminergic (H$_1$ receptors)
        Serotonergic (5-HT$_3$ receptors)
        Neurokinin-1 receptors

Agonists

        Steroids
        Cannabinoids

Dexamethasone has been shown to be an effective anti-emetic for the prophylaxis of PONV (LopezOlaondo *et al.* 1996). It is not used widely as yet, but it may be useful when initial anti-emetic therapy has failed. It has used successfully in combination with other anti-emetics (*vide infra*). The use of cannabinoids for nausea and vomiting associated with chemotherapy is well established (Dalzell *et al.* 1986) but there are no consistent data confirming efficacy for PONV (Lewis *et al.* 1994). Nabilone and dronabinol have been used, albeit with high incidence of side effects (Kumar *et al.* 2001).

Non-pharmacological methods

Acupuncture has been shown to be effective for the treatment of PONV and is reviewed in some detail in chapter 3. Vickers analysed 33 studies investigating acupuncture administered during GA ($n = 4$) or when awake ($n = 29$) (Vickers 1996). Clinical situations included PONV ($n = 21$), morning sickness ($n = 7$) and chemotherapy ($n = 5$). In those studies where acupuncture was administered to the awake patient ($n = 29$), 27 showed acupuncture to be effective. A meta-analysis of 19 controlled trials has shown that using non-pharmacological techniques (acupunture, electroacupuncture, acupoint stimulation, acupressure and transcutaneous electrical nerve stimulation) can reduce the incidence of early and late vomiting after surgery (Lee & Done 1999).

Failure of anti-emetic prophylaxis in a patient population

Clinical audit or simple clinical impression may indicate that the incidence of PONV in a certain population of patients is unacceptably high despite the administration of an anti-emetic drug. We now discuss the options available in this situation.

Organisational factors

This is a very common cause for the failure of anti-emetic prophylaxis in a group of patients, as well as in any individual patient (*vide supra*). These are discussed in detail in Chapter 8.

Choice of drug and dose

There is a wealth of literature about the efficacy of anti-emetics in the prophylaxis of PONV in many types of surgery. However, it is not possible to make conclusions about the relative efficacy of these drugs with respect to type of surgery. It would make sense to change the drug if the first choice medication was ineffective and this should be done taking into account the principles discussed above. The question of dose has been considered.

Combination therapy

If there are no organisational problems, and what was thought to be an appropriate drug in a suitable dose has proven ineffective, then combination therapy should be considered. Combining two anti-emetics with different sites of action could have an additive affect compared with single drug therapy. Currently, there is considerable interest in this in the literature. Some of the published studies do not allow direct comparison of each individual drug with the combination. In these studies, the combination group is not compared directly with groups receiving each of the two drugs used in combination. Many compare the combination with one other group only. In general, most have found combinations more efficacious than a single drug. The literature is supportive of the efficacy of anti-emetic combination for the prevention and treatment of PONV (ASA Task Force on Postanesthetic Care 2002; Heffernan & Rowbotham 2000).

Some of the studies investigating ondansetron droperidol combination are summarised in Table 5.6. One of the first was by Pueyo and colleagues who studied females undergoing intra-abdominal surgery (75% gynaecological). Anti-emetic therapy was given in a randomised double-blind manner at, and 12 h after, induction of anaesthesia. There were four groups: placebo then placebo, droperidol 2.5 mg then droperidol 1.25 mg, ondansetron 4 mg then placebo, droperidol 2.5 mg plus ondansetron 4 mg then droperidol 1.25 mg. Ondansetron and droperidol were superior to placebo but the combination was significantly more effective than monotherapy. For example, at 12 h, the incidence of nausea was 8% in the combination group compared with 28% and 40% in the droperidol and ondansetron groups, respectively. A similar pattern was observed up to 48 h post-operatively. The overall incidence of PONV remained 8% in the combination group compared with 40% and 44% in the droperidol

Table 5.6 Droperidol ondansetron combinations

Reference	Combinations	Surgery	Results
Pueyo et al. (1996)	Ondan, Drop	Major gynaecological	Improved
Wu et al. (2000)	Drop + Ondan	Laparoscopy	Improved
Wrench et al. (1996)	Ondan, Drop Drop + Ondan (Added to PCA)	Major gynaecological	Improved (first 12 h only)
Riley et al. (1998)	Drop Drop + Ondan	Major gynaecological	Improved
Klockgether Radke. et al. (1997)	Drop, Ondan Drop + Ondan	Paediatric Strabismus	No improvement
Shende et al. 2001	Drop, Ondan Drop + Ondan	Paediatric strabismus	Improvement

Ondan, ondansetron; Drop, droperidol.

and ondansetron groups, respectively. Similarly, the combination of droperidol 1.25 mg and ondansetron 4 mg resulted in significant reduction of the incidence of PONV in the first 24 hours in patients undergoing gynaecological laparoscopy (Wu *et al.* 2000)

The comparative efficacy of combinations of droperidol and ondansetron has been compared when given as a mixture within a patient-controlled analgesia (PCA) syringe. Wrench and colleagues investigated 60 patients undergoing gynaecological surgery and post-operative PCA (morphine 1 mg/ml) (Wrench *et al.* 1996). Patients were randomised to receive three anti-emetic regimens: (i) ondansetron 4 mg bolus plus ondansetron 8 mg per 60-ml syringe; (ii) droperidol 1.25 mg plus droperidol 3 mg per 60-ml syringe; (iii) a combination of both drugs as a bolus plus both drugs added to the syringe. There was a relatively low incidence of PONV in all groups in this study but at 12 h post-operatively the incidence of nausea in the combination group was 5% compared with 20 and 25% in the droperidol and ondansetron groups, respectively ($p < 0.05$).

Several studies have shown not only efficacy of dexamethasone for the prevention of PONV but also increased efficacy when used in combination with ondansetron, granisetron, tropisetron and droperidol (Table 5.7). For example, Splinter and Rhine (1998) gave children undergoing squint surgery one of two anti-emetic regimens in a randomised double-blind manner: ondansetron 150 µg/kg (maximum 8 mg) or ondansetron 50 µg/kg plus dexamethasone 150 µg/kg (maximum 8 mg). The design of this study was not ideal as discussed above but the incidence of vomiting at 24 h was 28% in the ondansetron group compared with 9% in the combination group. Furthermore, no children in the combination group vomited on the way home.

Table 5.7 Ondansetron–dexamethasone, granisetron–dexamethasone and tropisetron–dexamethasone combinations

Reference	Combinations	Surgery	Results
McKenzie *et al.* (1994)	Ondan Ondan + Dexameth	Major gynaecological	Improved
Lopezolaondo *et al.* (1996)	Ondan, Dexameth Ondan + Dexameth	Major gynaecological	Improved
Splinter & Rhine (1998)	Ondan Ondan + Dexameth	Paediatric Strabismus	Improved
Fujii *et al.* (2000)	Gran Gran + Dexameth	Laparoscopic cholecystectomy	Improved
Fujii *et al.* (1998)	Gran, Dexameth Gran + Dexameth	Middle ear surgery	Improved
Holt *et al.* (2000)	Tropis Tropis + Dexameth	Paediatric tonsillectomy	Improved

Ondan, ondasetron; Gran, granisetron; Dexameth, dexamethasone;Tropis, tropisetron.

The combination of granisetron and dexamethasone was superior to granisetron or dexamethasone alone in patients undergoing laparoscopic cholecystectomy and middle ear surgery (Fujji *et al.* 1998, 2000). Similarly, the combination of ondansetron 4 mg and cyclizine 50 mg reduced the incidence of vomiting and the severity of nausea for up to 24 hours after gynaecological laparoscopy when compared with ondansetron 4 mg alone (Ahmed *et al.* 2000).

Lopez-Olando and colleagues investigated patients undergoing major gynaecological surgery (LopezOlaondo *et al.* 1996) in a study of good design. Anti-emetics were given at induction of anaesthesia: placebo, ondansetron 4 mg, dexamethasone 8 mg or a combination of dexamethasone and ondansetron at the same doses. Both ondansetron and dexamethasone were significantly better than placebo but the combination was significantly more efficacious than all groups. For example, the incidence of nausea at 24 h was 48% in the ondansetron group and 40% in the dexamethasone group compared with 76% in the placebo group. The incidence of nausea in the combination group was only 12%.

Recent studies have focused attention on the use of dolasetron as part of combination anti-emetic regimens (Coloma *et al.* 2002; Sukhani *et al.* 2002; Piper *et al.* 2003) and clinical experience of this agent – recently introduced into the UK – is awaited with much interest.

The future of anti-emetic therapy

There is considerable potential for improving our success in preventing and treating PONV. This chapter and others have discussed several relevant areas. Perhaps, with the introduction of new drugs, the problem of the patient who has not responded to anti-emetic therapy will be infrequent. We live in hope. Perhaps a more appropriate way forward is to embrace the concept of balanced anti-emesis i.e. using several anti-emetics with different sites of action. This principle was implemented several years ago for post-operative pain relief.

References

Allen, A., Asgill, C.C., Pierce, D.M., Upward, J. & Zussman, B.D. (1994). Pharmacokinetics and tolerability of ascending intravenous doses of granisetron, a novel 5-HT3 antagonist, in healthy human subjects. *European Journal of Clinical Pharmacology* **46**, 159–162.

Ahmed, A.B., Hobbs, G.J. & Curran, J.P. (2000). Randomised, placebo-controlled trial of combination anti-emetic prophylaxis for day-case gynaecological laparoscopic surgery. *British Journal of Anaesthesia* **85**, 678–682.

American Society of Anesthesiology Task Force on Postanesthetic Care (2002). Practice guidelines for the postanesthetic care. *Anaesthesiology* **96**, 724–752.

Boxenbaum, H., Gillespie, T., Heck, K. & Hahne, W. (1993). Human dolasetron pharmacokinetics.2. Absorption and disposition following single-dose oral-administration to normal-male subjects. *Biopharmaceutics and Drug Disposition* **14**, 131–141.

Balfour, J.A.& Goa, K.L. (1997). Dolasetron – a review of its pharmacology and therapeutic potential in the management of nausea and vomiting induced by chemotherapy, radiotherapy or surgery. *Drugs* **54**, 273–298.

Coloma, M., White, P.F., Markowitz, S.D., *et al.* (2002). Dexamethasone in combination with dolasetron for prophylaxis in the ambulatory setting: effect on outcome after laparascopic cholecystectomy. *Anesthesiology* **96**, 1346–1350.

Cressman, W.A., Plostnieks, J. & Johnson, P.C. (1973). Absorption, metabolism and excretion of droperidol by human subjects following intramuscular and intravenous administration. *Anesthesiology* **38**, 363–369.

Dimmitt, D.C., Choo, Y.S., Martin, L.A., Arumugham, T., Hahne, W.F. & Weir, S.J. (1999). Intravenous pharmacokinetics and absolute oral bioavailability of dolasetron in healthy volunteers: Part 1. *Biopharmaceutics and Drug Disposition* **20**, 29–39.

Dalzell, A.M., Bartlett, H. & Lilleyman, J.S. (1986). Nabilone: an alternative anti-emetic for cancer chemotherapy. *Archives of Disease In Childhood* **61**, 502–505.

Fischler, M., Bonnet, F., Trang, H. *et al.* (1986). The pharmacokinetics of droperidol in anesthetized patients. *Anesthesiology* **64**, 486–489.

Fukuda, H., Koga, T., Furukawa, N., Nakamura, E. & Shiroshita, Y. (1999). The tachykinin NK1 receptor antagonist GR205171 abolishes the retching activity of neurons comprising the central pattern generator for vomiting in dogs. *Neuroscience Research* **33**, 25–32.

Fujii, Y., Saiton, Y., Tanaka, H. & Toyooka, H. (2000). Granisetron/dexamethasone combination for the prevention of postoperative nausea and vomiting after laparoscopic cholecystectomy. *European Journal of Anaesthesiology* **17**, 64–68.

Fujii, Y., Toyooka, H. & Tanaka, H. (1998). Prophylactic anti-emetic therapy with a combination of granisetron and dexamethasone in patients undergoing middle ear surgery. *British Journal of Anaesthesia* **81**, 754–756.

Griffin, D.S. & Baselt, R.C. (1984). Blood and urine concentrations of cyclizine by nitrogen-phosphorus gas-liquid chromatography. *Journal of Analytical Toxicology* **8**, 97–99.

Grunwald, Z., Torjman, M., Schieren, H. & Bartkowski, R.R. (1993). The pharmacokinetics of droperidol in anesthetized children. *Anesthesia and Analgesia* **76**, 1238–1242.

Gesztesi, Z., Scuderi, P.E., White, P. *et al.* (2000). Substance P (neurokinin-1) antagonist prevents postoperative vomiting after abdominal hysterectomy procedures. *Anaesthesiology* **93**, 931–937.

Harrington, R.A., Hamilton, C.W., Brogden, R.N., Linkewich, J.A., Romankiewicz, J.A. & Heel, R.C. (1983). Metoclopramide: An updated review of its pharmacological properties and clinical use. *Drugs* **25**, 451–494.

Henzi, I., Walder, B. & Tramer, M.R. (1999). Metoclopramide in the prevention of postoperative nausea and vomiting: A quantitative systematic review of randomised placebo controlled trials. *British Journal of Anaesthesia* **83**, 761–771.

Heffernan, A.M. & Rowbotham, D.J. (2000). Postoperative nausea and vomiting - time for balanced antiemesis? *British Journal of Anaesthesia* **85**, 675–677.

Holt, R., Rask, P., Coulthard, K.P. *et al.* (2000). Tropisetron plus dexamethasone is more effective than tropisetron alone for the prevention of postoperative nausea and vomiting in children undergoing tonsillectomy. *Paediatric Anaesthesia* **10**, 181–188.

Hamilton, D.L. (1998). Droperidol-ondansetron combination versus droperidol alone for postoperative control of emesis after total abdominal hysterectomy. *Journal of Clinical Anesthesia* **10**, 6–12.

Isah, A.O., Rawlins, M.D. & Bateman, D.N. (1992). The pharmacokinetics and effects of prochlorperazine in elderly female volunteers. *Age and Ageing* **21**, 27–31.

Kudoh, S., Okada, H., Miyazaki, R. *et al.* (1993). A phase I study of granisetron hydrochloride (2) - Pharmacokinetics of granisetron following single oral administration in healthy Japanese subjects. *Japanese Pharmacology and Therapeutics* **21**, 169–176.

Kumar, R.N., Chambers, W.N., Pertwee, R.G. (2001). Pharmacological actions and therapeutic uses of cannabis and cannabinoids. *Anaesthesia* **56**, 1059–1068.

KlockgetherRadke, A., Neumann, S., Neumann, P., Braun, U. & Muhlendyck, H. (1997). Ondansetron, droperidol and their combination for the prevention of post-operative vomiting in children. *European Journal of Anaesthesiology* **14**, 362–367.

Lewis, I.H., Campbell, D.N. & Barrowcliffe, M.P. (1994). Effect of nabilone on nausea and vomiting after total abdominal hysterectomy. *British Journal of Anaesthesia* **73**, 244–246.

Lee, A. & Done, M.L. (1999). The use of nonpharmacological techniques to prevent postoperative nausea and vomiting: a meta-analysis. *Anesthesia and Analgesia* **88**, 1362–1369.

LopezOlaondo, L., Carrascosa, F., Pueyo, F.J., Monedero, P., Busto, N., Saez, A. (1996). Combination of ondansetron and dexamethasone in the prophylaxis of postoperative nausea and vomiting. *British Journal of Anaesthesia* **76**, 835–840.

McKenzie, R., Kovac, A., O'Connor, T. *et al.* (1993). Comparison of ondansetron versus placebo to prevent postoperative nausea and vomiting in women undergoing ambulatory gynecologic surgery. *Anesthesiology* **78**, 21–28.

Marshall, S.I., & Chung, F. (1999). Discharge criteria and complications after ambulatory surgery. *Anesthesia and Analgesia* **88**, 508–517.

McKenzie, R., Tantisira, B., Karambelkar, D.J., Riley, T.J. & Abdelhady, H. (1994). Comparison of ondansetron with ondansetron plus dexamethasone in the prevention of postoperative nausea and vomiting. *Anesthesia and Analgesia* **79**, 961–964.

Nahata, M.C., Ford, C. & Ruymann, F.B. (1992). Pharmacokinetics and safety of prochlorperazine in pediatric-patients receiving cancer-chemotherapy. *Journal of Clinical Pharmacy and Therapeutics* **17**, 121–123.

Piper, S.N., Triem, J.G., Rohm, K.D., Kranke, P., Maleck, W.H. & Boldt, J. (2003). Prevention of postoperative nausea and vomiting. Randomised comparison of dolasetron versus dolasetron plus dexamethasone. *Anaesthesist* **52**, 120–126.

Pueyo, F.J., Carrascosa, F., Lopez, L., Iribarren, M.J., GarciaPedrajas, F. & Saez, A. (1996). Combination of ondansetron and droperidol in the prophylaxis of postoperative nausea and vomiting. *Anesthesia and Analgesia* **83**, 117–122.

Ross-Lee, L.M., Hooper, W.D. & Bochner, F. (1981). Single-dose pharmacokinetics of metoclopramide. *European Journal of Pharmacology* **20**, 465–471.

Roila, F. & Delfavero, A. (1995). Ondansetron clinical pharmacokinetics. *Clinical Pharmacokinetics* **29**, 95–109.

Rowbotham, D.J. (1992). Current management of postoperative nausea and vomiting. *British Journal of Anaesthesia* **69**, 46S–59S.

Riley, T.J., McKenzie, R., Trantisira, B.R. & Hamilton, D.L. (1998). Droperidol-ondansetron combination versus droperidol alone for postoperative control of emesis after total abdominal hysterectomy. *Journal of Clinical Anesthesia* **10**, 6–12.

Shende, D., Bharti, N., Kathirvel, S. & Madan, R. (2001). Combination of droperidol and ondansetron reduces PONV after paediatric strabismus surgery more than single drug therapy. *Acta Anaesthesiologica Scandanavia* **45**, 756–760.

Splinter, W.M. & Rhine, E.J. (1998). Low-dose ondansetron with dexamethasone more effectively decreases vomiting after strabismus surgery in children than does high-dose ondansetron. *Anesthesiology* **88**, 72–75.

Sukhani, R., Pappas, A.L., Lurie, J., Hotaling, A.J., Park, A. & Fluder, E. (2002). Ondansetron and dolasetron provide equivalent vomiting control after ambulatory tonsillectomy in dexamethasone-pretreated children. *Anesthesia and Analgesia* **95**, 1230–1235.

Taylor, W.B. & Bateman, D.N. (1987). Preliminary studies of the pharmacokinetics and pharmacodynamics of prochlorperazine in healthy-volunteers. *British Journal of Clinical Pharmacology* **23**, 137–142.

Vickers, A.J. (1996). Can acupuncture have specific effects on health? A systematic review of acupuncture anti-emetic trials. *Journal of the Royal Society of Medicine* **89**, 303–311.

Walker, R.B. & Kanfer, I. (1996). Pharmacokinetics of cyclizine following intravenous administration to human volunteers. *European Journal of Pharmaceutical Sciences* **4**, 301–306.

Wu, O., Belo, S.E. & Koutsoukos, G. (2000). Additive anti-emetic efficacy of prophylactic ondansetron with droperidol in out-patient gynaecological laparoscopy. *Canadian Journal of Anaesthesia* **47**, 529–536.

Wrench, L.J., Ward, J.H., Walder, A.D. & Hobbs, G.J. (1996). The prevention of postoperative nausea and vomiting using a combination of ondansetron and droperidol. *Anaesthesia* **51**, 776–778.

Chapter 6

Pharmaceutical considerations in the preparation and administration of anti-emetic agents

Philip Howard

Introduction

About 56% (Anon. 1993) of the four million patients that have operations in UK hospitals every year (Anon. 1998) are given anti-emetics to treat or prevent PONV. Of these, most are prescribed as intramuscular, 'p.r.n.' injections on ward areas or are given intravenous boluses or infusions within the operating-theatre complex. Anaesthetists will predominantly use the intravenous route and nurses the intramuscular route. This procedure is so routine that probably very little thought goes into the process. However, many of issues are involved in this process, and these will be discussed in this chapter.

The main elements of the process and their related issues can be divided as follows:

- *Selection of anti-emetics*
    - product liability for licensed drugs
    - liability for unlicensed medicines
    - patient consent

- *Preparation of anti-emetics*
    - particulate contamination and its prevention
    - microbiological contamination and its prevention
    - labelling of syringes
    - compatibility of admixtures
    - stability of infusions.

- *Administration of anti-emetics*
    - route and adverse effects
    - rate of injection.

Selection of anti-emetics

Product liability for licensed medicines

The initial selection of an anti-emetic should be based upon four main considerations:

- Safety
- Efficacy
- Cost effectiveness
- Product license of the anti-emetic

The Strict Liability Consumer Protection Act 1987 states that a manufacturer is liable for untoward events so long as the product was used according to its license and stored appropriately before use. When using a medicine for an unlicensed use the manufacturer will retain liability for quality, but the user retains clinical liability – usually the NHS Trust and prescriber. The same applies for an unlicensed medicine.

A European Council directive of 1987 made it a legal obligation for all medicines to be supplied with a patient information leaflet. This came into effect in the UK in 1999. In 2001, the Department of Health published a document on Consenting Patients. It gave direction that all patients or carers must give consent before being examined, receiving care or treatment. Consent can be written, verbal of non-verbal.

Based on this document, many Trusts have taken the decision that the use of unlicensed medicines or some unlicensed uses of licensed medicines should have an information leaflet for the patients to read before obtaining consent.

A 2002 survey of surgical & theatres pharmacists, showed that around 10% of Trusts or Hospitals are still using droperidol despite it being withdrawn by the UK manufacturers. Those hospitals still using the products were importing either a Canadian or US licensed product. It is, however, unlikely that droperidol will remain licensed within these countries for much longer. None of the hospitals were consenting patients before use.

Licensed routes for anti-emetics

Drug	po	iv	im	sc	rectal
Cyclizine	yes	yes	yes	no	n/a
Dolasetron	yes	yes	no	no	n/a
Droperidol	no	no	no	no	n/a
Granisetron	yes	yes	no	no	n/a
Metoclopramide	yes	yes	yes	no	n/a
Ondansetron	yes	yes	yes	no	yes
Prochlorperazine	yes	no	yes	no	yes

Preparation of anti-emetics
Particulate contamination in intravenous medication

All injectable medication contains particulate contamination; this can be classified into intrinsic and extrinsic contamination, depending on its origin (see Table 6.1).

Table 6.1 Sources of particulate contamination

Intrinsic	Extrinsic
Metal	Rubber
Glass	Plastic
Cotton	Glass
Barium sulphate	Cotton
	Precipitates

Intrinsic contamination

Intrinsic contamination arises during the manufacturing process, transport and storage. In 1973, the British Pharmacopoeia (BP) introduced limits for the particulate matter allowed in large-volume fluids. These limits were not based on any clinical evidence of the harmful effects of infused particles. Filtration during the manufacturing process allowed these limits to be easily met. However, the BP did not set limits for particulate matter for small volume fluids (less than 100 ml) or freeze-dried powders. The United States Pharmacopoeia (USP) set limits for both large- and small-volume fluids (see Table 6.2).

Studies into the intrinsic particulate contamination of small-volume fluids showed that there is large variation in total particle counts between different drugs, but also between different batches of the same drug (Backhouse *et al.* 1987). More astonishingly, the particulate matter in freeze-dried drugs after reconstitution in a carrier fluid was found to be up to ten times more than those drugs already in solution.

Intrinsic contamination can also be generated by interaction between the drug and its container during transportation and storage.

Extrinsic contamination

Extrinsic contamination is generated through the various manipulations involved in administering drugs and infusions. When an ampoule is opened, glass particles are released. Many of these are visible, i.e. >40 μm, but many others are not. The glass particles fall back into the ampoule and are drawn up through the needle into the syringe (Shaw & Lyall 1985) A 0.2 μm end-line filter has been shown to eliminate these particles (Sabon *et al.* 1989). Cores of rubber bungs can be released when a needle pierces a bung. Particles of plastic are also released from administration equipment, such as giving sets and syringes (Taylor 1982). The introduction by some pharmaceutical companies of the plastic (polypropylene) flexi-amp is progress towards fewer particles, especially when the use of filters outside of intensive care areas is minimal in many hospitals.

If drugs are physically incompatible, they may precipitate out into solution generating many more particles.

Table 6.2 Particulate matter standards

British and European Pharmacopoeias		
Large-volume parenterals (>100 ml)		
No more than	1000/ml	>2 μm
No more than	100/ml	>5 μm

United States Pharmacopoeia		
Large-volume parenterals (>100 ml)		
No more than	50/ml	<10 μm
No more than	5/ml	<5 μm
Small-volume parenterals (<100 ml)		
No more than	1000 per container	<25 μm
No visible particles should be present		

Table 6.3 Size of particulate matter

	μm
Blood set filter	200
Human hair	120
Visual limits	80
Industry standard filter	15
Blood corpuscle	7.5
Small blood capillary	5
Chylomicron	4
Candida (yeast)	2
Spores	1.2+
Bacteria	0.2+
Virus	0.1

Clinical consequences of particulate infusion

The clinical effects of particulate matter can be divided into two parts: local effects and systemic effects. Local effects involve irritation of the vein at the cannula entry site (phlebitis). Systemic effects result from the particles being removed from the circulation by various organs, especially the lungs.

Phlebitis

Phlebitis is a common adverse effect of intravenous therapy and the effects can last for many weeks after therapy. Up to 50% of patients get phlebitis (Falchuk *et al.* 1985). Patient groups where intravenous access is difficult can have a lot of discomfort from regular cannulae changes that are short-lived because of phlebitis.

Many factors have been implicated in infusion phlebitis. Infection is often thought to be the main cause, but is rare with less than 1% of catheter tips being successfully cultured (Francombe 1998). It appears that particulate contamination is the major culprit, but the use of microfilters can reduce the incidence of phlebitis by 50% (Allcutt *et al.* 1983). Table 6.4 shows common causes of infusion-related phlebitis.

Systemic effects

Particles with a diameter of 7–12 μm that are injected into the systemic circulation are usually removed by the pulmonary capillary bed. Larger particles become trapped and undergo phagocytosis, if biodegradable; if not, a granuloma is formed, surrounded by mononucleocytes and foreign body giant cells with a fibrous sheath around the outside. The use of end-line filters has shown a lower ESR and WCC (De Luca *et al.* 1976).

Accidental air emboli

These can form in many different ways. Intravenous fluid on warming up from cool storage can release small bubbles. Also, additional bubbles can arise from priming. Infusion of non-collapsible containers or accidental disconnection can also result in air entering the circulation. Fatalities can occur dependent upon the volume of air administered or the rate of infusion (Marshall & Lloyd 1987). The use of infusion pumps and 0.2 μm air venting filters can prevent this adverse effect.

Microbiological contamination

This also can be separated into intrinsic and extrinsic contamination. Intrinsic contamination is microbiological contamination during the manufacturing and transport process. This is very rare. Guidelines are in place for intravenous fluids and the giving sets that they flow to be changed every 24 hours, where possible, to prevent repetition of hospital-acquired sepsis related to contaminated intravenous fluids (Macmillan 1972).

Table 6.4 Possible causes of infusion-related phlebitis cannula type

Infusion pH
Infusion tonicity
Location of IV site
Duration of infusion
Infection
Particulate matter

Table 6.5 *In vivo* effects of particulate contamination

Systemic effects	Local effects
Inflammation	Phlebitis
Granulomata	
Thrombi	
Lung lesions	
ARDS	
Multi-organ failure	

Extrinsic contamination is the result of manipulations of the intravenous administration systems while in use. The usual sources of infection are three-way taps, injection ports and connecting taps (Clayton *et al.* 1985). When a needle pierces an injection port, a warm meniscus of fluid is left behind. This is an ideal environment for bacterial growth. Any subsequent injections through the port will also inject any inoculate into the patient. The rate of in-use contamination of intravenous fluids ranges from 0 to 30% with an average value of 3% (Marshall & Lloyd 1987). It has also been shown that Gram-negative bacteria can grow to large numbers within 24 hours in simple intravenous infusions at room temperature (e.g. *Klebsiella* sp. 10^5 per millilitre in 5% glucose with 24 hours) (Maki *et al.* 1971). Total parenteral nutrition is probably the most ideal growth medium, and many hospitals insist on a dedicated IV line for total parenteral nutrition (Ng *et al.* 1989; Twum-Danso *et al.* 1989). It has been demonstrated that 0.2 μm filters are required, as 0.45 μm filters have been penetrated by certain bacteria (Holmes *et al.* 1980). Clinically significant nosocomial bacteraemia occurs less in a surgical intensive care unit (ICU) with the use of 0.2 μm filters (Quercia *et al.* 1986). End-line IV filters need to be changed every 24 hours as Gram-negative bacteria start to autolyse and release significant amounts of endotoxin. Endotoxin infusion results in pyrogenic, toxic and inflammatory reactions (Wardle 1986). There are some negatively charged filters that can trap the positively charged endotoxins for periods of up to 96 hours (Baumgartner *et al.* 1986).

Problems with filters

Filters are ideal for preventing particulate and microbiological contamination from reaching the systemic circulation, but they can have drawbacks. Most drugs can be filtered, so long as they are completely soluble. Agents that are not filterable are those drugs formulated as suspensions or emulsions or those which are not fully dissolved in their solvent. Of the agents used or considered anti-emetic, propofol is the only one. Propofol is a fat emulsion and should not be passed through a filter smaller than 5 μm. Also of importance is the fact that many blood constituents are too large to go through 0.2 μm filters. Red blood cells are 7.5 μm and platelets are 2–4 μm in diameter so standard 0.2 μm filters cannot be used when administering these.

The problem of drugs binding to filters (sorption) has been studied extensively (Trissell 1998). Most drugs delivered at high concentrations or fast-flow rates through administration sets will not bind significantly. Most end-line filters have a dead space so anti-emetics that need to reach the systemic circulation quickly will need a flush after administration.

Stability of infusions

The Committee for Proprietary Medicinal Products at the European Agency for the Evaluation of Medicinal Products (EMEA) have produced guidance in 1999 on the maximum shelf-life for sterile products for human use after first opening or following reconstitution. The guidance was designed to make manufacturers provide instructions to the user on storage times and conditions once a sterile product has been opened. They require the manufacturer to state for preparations for infusion or injection from unpreserved sterile products:

- chemical and physical in-use stability has been demonstrated for x hours/days at y °C
- from a microbiological point of view, the product should be used immediately. If not used immediately, in-use storage times and conditions prior to use are the responsibility of the user and would normally not be longer than 24 hours at 2–8 °C, unless reconstitution/dilution has taken place in a controlled and validated aseptic conditions.

Labelling of anti-emetics

It is recommended that anti-emetics be prepared immediately before use (Anon 1998). If anti-emetics are drawn up within the anaesthetic room in advance to give to a patient, they should be clearly labelled. Most injections are clear, colourless solutions which are difficult to distinguish, so can easily be mixed up without correct or any labelling. There have been many fatalities associated with not labelling syringes (Cousins & Upton 1998). The operating theatres seem to be the worst affected for unlabelled syringes, often with the anaesthetist and ODA preparing drugs and leaving them unlabelled on the anaesthetic room bench (Cousins & Upton 1998).

Compatibility of admixtures

With the poor outcomes using monotherapy for anti-emetics, the use of dual or more combinations will become more common. Also, there will be clinical situations when there is a need for anti-emetics to be added to solutions or mixed with other drugs – for example:

- to reduce the number of intramuscular injections a patient receives (e.g. combining an opioid with an anti-emetic);
- when incorporating an anti-emetic into a patient-controlled analgesic system (e.g. morphine and droperidol syringes);
- in ICUs when drugs and infusions come together on a three-way tap before entering the patient. If any of these infusions or drugs are incompatible, they may come out of solution to form a precipitate of solid particles which may be gelatinous, crystalline or granular in nature. The end-line filter will protect the patient but the filter will be occluded.

Drug stability and compatibility are crucial elements in drug delivery. There are a number of reasons for physical drug incompatibility, including:

- imbalance of drugs dissolved in complex co-solvents when added to other solutions;
- drugs that are weak acids or bases are formulated at high or low pH values to keep them in solution. If the pH changes markedly on adding to another solution, the drug may come out of solution;
- precipitation due to formation of salts that are relatively insoluble (e.g. calcium and phosphates);
- formation of insoluble complexes with large organic anions and actions (e.g. heparin and aminoglycosides).

Sorption phenomena can also be subclassified into two sorts:

- adsorption of a drug to the surface of a container (e.g. glass or plastics in bags, administration sets or filters). This is only important if a drug is given in low concentrations or small amounts as the amount adsorbed may be significant. At higher amounts or concentrations, saturation of binding sites occurs and is less significant;
- absorption into the matrix of plastic containers and administration sets, especially PVC, is another source of drug loss for lipid soluble drugs in solution. Polypropylene and polyethylene do not have the same problem as they contain no or little phthalate plasticisers.

Compatibility of drugs is often classified into four distinct areas:

* the drug in a solution for infusion;
* the drug added to another drug in a solution for infusion;
* the drug added to another drug in a syringe for infusion;
* drugs mixing at a Y site before entering a patient.

The appendix to this chapter, on pages 94–105, outlines some of the compatibility issues for parenteral anti-emetics in use in the UK. Only drugs commonly used in combination are included. More detailed information regarding drug compatibility is available from standard texts such as Trissell (1998).

General guidelines on admixtures

To minimise risk with the mixing of anti-emetics with other agents, it is better to publicise a small range of compatible agents in the ICUs, theatres and wards. This is already provided by some medical filter companies (e.g. Pall Medical Ltd).

The newer agents, such as ondansetron, seem to have a lot of compatibility work undertaken on them, which is useful.

Administration of anti-emetics

In the post-operative period, anti-emetics are usually given by two routes: intravenous or intramuscular. The intravenous route is the better of the two routes because of its bioavailability and speed of onset. The intramuscular route is problematic and should only be used in situations when nurses are not approved to give drugs by the intravenous route. Measures should be taken within hospitals to enable nurses to give anti-emetics into running fluids or directly into cannulae.

Intramuscular route

This route is complicated by the variable bioavailability of the drugs administered. It can often be slow, erratic or incomplete. The site of injection also affects the speed of absorption: fastest from the deltoid muscle and slowest from the gluteal muscles. Blood flow to the muscles is reduced in circulatory collapse or if cardiac output is low and can thus reduce absorption even more (Aronson 1995). Although it is common practice to swab the injection site before injection, it is probably unnecessary (Dann 1969).

Adverse effects do arise from intramuscular injections. The most common being skin reactions at the site of injection. Those agents whose pH differs markedly from the surrounding tissue, and which are or contain chemical irritants are the most troublesome. Incorrect administration technique is usually the main cause (Uchegbu & Florence 1996). A small number (0.4%) of patients complain of persistent pain, erythema, a weal, induration, subcutaneous fat nodules, haematoma, bleeding, or abscess. These are more common in children (23%). Pain in the muscle can also occur, and is partly related to the volume of the injection, which should generally be no more than 2 ml into the arm or thigh, but up to 5 ml into gluteus maximus (Hipwell *et al.* 1984). Local muscle damage is common. A rise in serum creatine kinase occurs and increases with the volume and concentration of the solution injected. It is not known whether the drug or diluent is the main cause. Patients who are anticoagulated or receiving thrombolysis should not receive intramuscular injections.

Of the anti-emetics that cause injection-site complications, prochlorperazine (0.1%) seems to be the most common, and promethazine has been implicated. These were probably linked to the difference in pH (Greenblatt & Allen 1978).

Intravenous route

A number of different problems arise with the intravenous route, including:

- intravenous delivery devices, such as patient-controlled analgesia pumps that sometimes contain anti-emetics as well as opioids, can malfunction (Whipple *et al.* 1994);
- there may be particulate contamination (see above);
- there may be microbiological contamination (see above);
- problems with preservatives used in intravenous delivery systems – deaths have been reported in neonates and children from metabolic acidosis from benzoic alcohol preservatives (these are not used in any anti-emetics);
- solubilisers used in intravenous injections have caused anaphylactic reactions, other hypersensitivity reactions such as hyperventilation, hypoxia and pruritus, and thrombophlebitis. Again these are not used in any anti-emetic agents. Propofol was formulated in cremaphor but is no longer. Pain can still be a problem in the new formulation – and propofol is often mixed with lidocaine to overcome this (Anon 1998b) – but it could be due to glass fragments (Driscoll *et al.* 1997).

Oral route

This route is often not appropriate for the treatment of PONV. Tablets are likely to be vomited back. The introduction of 'Melt' tablets allows the patient to swallow the tablet without water. However, the tablets are still absorbed from the small bowel so absorption is not necessarily quicker.

Rectal route

The rectal route can be used for the administration of anti-emetics. The absorption can be erratic, incomplete and slow dependant on the agent used. The rectal mucosa is also sensitive to irritants. However, there are some advantages to this route. Only 50% of any drug absorbed by this route goes straight to the liver, so the remainder avoid the first pass metabolism by the liver. It can also be useful where parenteral administration is not appropriate.

Subcutaneous route

No anti-emetics routinely used for the treatment and prevention of PONV are licensed by this route. The route is gaining popularity with the use of indwelling subcutaneous catheters. Absorption from subcutaneous tissue can be fast enough to be effective so long as the patient is not too fat. Certain anti-emetics are not appropriate by this route because their pH or other chemicals in the solution, i.e. Prochlorperazine or promethazine.

Rate of administration

Rate of administration of intravenous injections and infusions is important. Most anti-emetics are given as a slow intravenous injection to reduce the risk of damage by high concentrations of drug at the site of injection. Most anti-emetics are formulated to an acidic pH. Some of the newer 5-HT$_3$ antagonists are given as intravenous infusions to further lower the risk of venous irritation.

The directions for the rate of administration suggested in the summary of product characteristics or data sheet for a drug (Anon 1998b) should always be followed by the nurse or anaesthetist giving the drug to prevent unwanted side-effects. At a ward level, the ward pharmacist can endorse the administration directions in the relevant box of the prescription card.

Conclusions

Ideally, all anti-emetics given intravenously should pass through an end-line filter to prevent particulate or microbial contamination from entering the patient. Anti-emetics should only be drawn up immediately before use, or labelled clearly. Anti-emetics should not be mixed with other agents, unless compatibility has been proven. The intravenous route should be used in preference to the intramuscular route for anti-emetic administration, if the oral route is not an option.

Appendix

Cyclizine (Valoid) (Anon 1998b)

Presentation: 50 mg tablets or 50 mg in 1 ml ampoules
Administration: oral, intramuscular or intravenous injection. The intravenous
injection should be given slowly, with only minimal withdrawal of blood from the
syringe (Anon. 1998)
pH: from 3.3 to 3.7 (Trissell 1998)
Stability: cyclizine injection is a colourless solution which should be protected
from light. A yellow tint may develop during storage but does not indicate a potency
loss. Cyclizine lactate is incompatible with any solution with a pH of 6.8 or greater.
Cyclizine has an aqueous solubility of 8 mg/ml. More concentrated solutions may
produce crystals within 24 hours (Trissell 1998)
Excipients: injection: lactic acid, water for injection
            tablets: lactose, potato starch, acacia, magnesium stearate,
                 purified water
There has been very little work done on the compatibility of cyclizine with other
agents with the exception of agents used in palliative care.
Compatibility (Trissell 1998)
Solution compatibility:
        Compatible: glucose 5% and water for injection
        Incompatible: sodium chloride 0.9%

Drugs compatible with cyclizine in a syringe for 24 hours:
        Compatible: diamorphine (dependent on concentration), diamorphine plus
        haloperidol (dependent on conc.), haloperidol, morphine (Bradley 1996),
        methadone (Dhami *et al.* 1995), ranitidine (Parker 1985)
        Incompatible: probably all drugs containing chloride ions (e.g.
        metoclopramide, granisetron, ondansetron, tropesetron, chlorpromazine)

Dexamethasone Sodium Phosphate (Anon 1998)

Presentation: 0.5 mg and 2 mg tablets, and 8 mg/2 ml ampoule
Administration: The injection can be given intravenously undiluted over one to several minutes or by continuous or intermittent infusion. It can be also be given by intramuscular injection
pH: from 7 to 8.5
Stability: the ampoules should be protected from light and freezing
Sorption: dexamethasone does not undergo significant absorption in PVC bags or tubing, cellulose burette chambers or in polypropylene or polythene syringes. It is not affected by 5 μm steel filters, 0.22 μm or 0.45 μm cellulose ester membrane or 0.22 μm polycarbonate filters
Excipients: nil
Compatibility (Trissell 1998)
Solution compatibility: dexamethasone is compatible with sodium chloride 0.9% and glucose 5% (see above)

Additive compatibility with dexamethasone:
  Compatible: granisetron, ondansetron, prochlorperazine
  Incompatible: diphenhydramine plus lorazepam plus metoclopramide

Drugs compatible with dexamethasone in a syringe for 24 hours:
  Compatible: granisetron, metoclopramide, ondansetron
  Incompatible: not known

Y site injection compatibility with dexamethasone:
  Compatible: granisetron, heparin, lorazepam, morphine, ondansetron, pethidine, propofol
  Incompatible: ciprofloxacin, midazolam

Dolasetron (Anzemet)

Presentation: 50 mg and 200 mg tablets, 12.5 mg in 1 ml ampoules and 100 mg in 5 ml ampoules

Administration: oral or intravenous injection. The intravenous injection can be injected over 30 seconds or diluted to 50 ml in normal saline, 5% dextrose or other compatible intravenous fluids and infused over a period of 30 seconds to 15 minutes

pH: 3.1–3.8

Stability: dilutions of intravenous fluids should be used immediately after preparation. If storage cannot be avoided, the maximum storage time for dilutions is 24 hours at 2–8C

Excipients: injection: Mannitol for injection, sodium acetate trihydrate, glacial acetic acid, water for injection

tablets: Lactose, pregelatinised starch, croscarmellose sodium, magnesium stearate

Compatibility

Solution compatibility:

Compatible: 5% glucose, 0.9% sodium chloride, 10% mannitol, compound sodium lactate, 0.18% sodium chloride/4% glucose

Drug compatibility:

Compatible: Hextend (Trissell 2003) Cimetidene (Dimmitt 1999)

Droperidol (Droleptan) (Anon 1998b)

Presentation: 10 mg tablets, 1 mg/ml liquid, and 10 mg/2 ml ampoule
Administration: the injection can be given intramuscularly or slow intravenous injection or intermittent or continuous intravenous infusion
pH: from 3 to 3.8
Stability: droperidol should be stored at room temperature and from light
Sorption: there is no problem with droperidol in PVC bags of sodium chloride 0.9% and 5% glucose solution, but sorption does take place in Ringer's solution
Excipients: mannitol, lactic acid
Compatibility (Trissell 1998)
Solution compatibility: droperidol is compatible with sodium chloride 0.9%, glucose 5% solution and Ringer's solution.

Additive compatibility with droperidol:
    Compatible: not known
    Incompatible: not known

Drugs compatible with droperidol in a syringe for 24 hours:
    Compatible: chlorpromazine, fentanyl, metoclopramide, pethidine, midazolam, morphine, nalbuphine, pentazocine, prochlorperazine, promethazine, hyoscine hydrobromide
    Incompatible: not known

Y site injection compatibility with droperidol:
    Compatible: aztreonam, granisetron, hydrocortisone, metoclopramide, morphine sulphate, potassium chloride, propofol
    Incompatible: heparin, tazocin

Granisetron (Kytril) (Anon 1998b)

Presentation: 1 mg and 2 mg tablets, 1 mg/5 ml liquid, and 1 mg/1 ml and
3 mg/1 ml vials
Administration: the injection can be given intravenously after dilution to 1 mg/5 ml
over 30 seconds or by intravenous infusion after dilution to 20–50 ml with sodium
chloride 0.9% or glucose 5% over five minutes
pH: from 4.7 to 7.3 (Trissell 1998)
Stability: granisetron should be stored at 30 °C or less and protected from freezing
and light. It is stable to pH changes. It is stable for 24 hours after dilution. Storage
conditions vary between presentations (see Summary of Product Characteristics –
Roche Products Ltd).
Excipients: none
Compatibility (Trissell 1998)
Solution compatibility: granisetron is compatible with water for injection, sodium
chloride 0.9% and glucose 5% solution, sodium chloride 0.18% and glucose 4%,
Hartman's solution, sodium lactate infusion, mannitol 10%

Additive compatibility with granisetron:
    Compatible: dexamethasone
    Incompatible: not known

Drugs compatible with granisetron in a syringe for 24 hours:
    Compatible: not known
    Incompatible: not known

Y site injection compatibility with granisetron:
    Compatible: aztreonam, buprenorphine, most commonly used UK
    cephalosporins, chlorpromazine, ciprofloxacin, dobutamine, dopamine,
    droperidol, haloperidol, heparin, hydrocortisone, lorazepam,
    metoclopramide, metronidazole, morphine sulphate, nalbuphine,
    pethidine, piperacillin, potassium chloride, prochlorperazine,
    promethazine, propofol, tazocin, vancomycin
    Incompatible: not known

Haloperidol (Anon 1998)

Presentation: 0.5 mg capsules, 1.5 mg, 5 mg, 10 mg and 20 mg tablets, 1 mg/ml and 2 mg/ml liquid, and 5 mg/1 ml, 10 mg/2 ml and 20 mg/2 ml ampoule
Administration: the injection can be given intramuscularly, subcutaneously or by intravenous injection and infusion
pH: from 3 to 3.6
Stability: haloperidol should be stored at room temperature and protected from light. Do not freeze or keep at temperatures above 40 °C
Excipients: lactic acid
Compatibility (Trissell 1998)
Solution compatibility: haloperidol is compatible in sodium chloride 0.9% and glucose 5% solution at low concentrations, but incompatible at high concentrations especially in sodium chloride 0.9%.

Additive compatibility with haloperidol:
       Compatible: not known
       Incompatible: not known

Drugs compatible with haloperidol in a syringe for 24 hours:
       Compatible: cyclizine (WFI or glucose 5% solution), diamorphine (dependent on concentration)
       Incompatible: ketorolac, morphine

Y site injection compatibility with haloperidol:
       Compatible: aztreonam, dobutamine, dopamine, glyceryl trinitrate, granisetron, midazolam, ondansetron, noradrenaline, phenylephrine, propofol
       Incompatible: heparin, tazocin

Metoclopramide (Maxolon) (Anon 1998b)

Presentation: 10 mg tablets, 5 g/5 ml oral solution, 10 mg/2 ml ampoule, and 100 mg/20 ml vial

Administration: the injection can be given intramuscularly or intravenously undiluted as 10 mg doses over 1 to 2 minutes or by intravenous dilution over 15 minutes after further dilution to 50 ml to 100 ml for larger doses, or to 500 ml and given over 8 to 12 hours

pH: from 3.6 to 6.5

Stability: metoclopramide should be stored at room temperature. It should not be frozen. It is stable over a pH range of 2 to 9. It is also photosensitive, but dilute solutions do not need to be protected from light. Discoloured solutions should be discarded

Excipients: sodium metabisulphite

Compatibility (Trissell 1998)

Solution compatibility: metoclopramide is compatible with most commonly used solutions

Additive compatibility with metoclopramide:
> **Compatible**: morphine sulphate, potassium chloride
> **Incompatible**: erythromycin

Drugs compatible with metoclopramide in a syringe for 24 hours:
> **Compatible**: dexamethasone, diamorphine, droperidol, fentanyl, hyoscine hydrobromide, methotrimeprazine, midazolam, morphine, pentazocine, pethidine, prochlorperazine, promazine, promethazine
> **Incompatible**: not known

Y site injection compatibility with ondansetron:
> **Compatible**: aztreonam, ciprofloxacin, droperidol, granisetron, heparin, morphine sulphate, ondansetron, pethidine, propofol, tazocin
> **Incompatible**: not known

Ondansetron (Zofran) (Anon 1998b)

Presentation: 4 mg and 8 mg tablets, 4 mg/5 ml syrup, 16 mg suppositories and 4 mg/2 ml and 8 mg/4 ml ampoule, 4 mg/2 ml and 8 mg/4 ml plastic (polypropylene) flexi-amps
Administration: the injection can be given intramuscularly or intravenously undiluted over at least 30 seconds and preferably over two to five minutes or over 15 minutes after further dilution with 50 ml of sodium chloride 0.9% or glucose 5%
pH: from 3.3 to 4
Stability: ondansetron is a stable solution. It should be stored at room temperature or refrigerated and protected from light. It is, however, stable for one month in daylight. It is also stable for up to one week when diluted with compatible solutions. Precipitation has been reported if combined with alkaline drugs. Ondansetron is not affected by in line 0.2 μm filters
Excipients: citric acid monohydrate, sodium citrate
Compatibility (Trissell 1998)
Solution compatibility: ondansetron is compatible with most commonly used solutions for up to a week

Additive compatibility with ondansetron:
> **Compatible**: dexamethasone (G5W & NS), morphine sulphate (NS), pethidine (NS)
> **Incompatible**: not known

Drugs compatible with ondansetron in a syringe for 24 hours:
> **Compatible**: dexamethasone (Trissell 1998), alfentanil, atropine, droperidol, fentanyl, glycopyrrolate, metoclopramide, midazolam, morphine, neostigmine, pethidine, and propofol (Stewart *et al.* 1998)
> **Incompatible**: not known

Y site injection compatibility with ondansetron:
> **Compatible**: aztreonam, most commonly used UK cephalosporins, chlorpromazine, dexamethasone, diphenhydramine, droperidol, haloperidol, heparin, hydrocortisone, hydromorphone, metoclopramide, morphine sulphate, pethidine, potassium chloride, prochlorperazine, promethazine, tazocin
> **Incompatible**: ampicillin, lorazepam, piperacillin

Prochlorperazine (Stemetil) (Anon 1998b)

Presentation: prochlorperazine is available as 5 mg and 25 mg tablets, 3 mg buccal tablets, 5 mg/5 ml syrup, 5 mg effervescent sachets, 5 mg and 25 mg suppositories and 12.5 mg/1 ml ampoule

Administration: the injection can be given intramuscularly deep into the upper outer quadrant of the buttock. It can be given undiluted as a slow intravenous injection at a rate not exceeding 5 mg/min to prevent local irritation. An intravenous infusion of 20 mg prochlorperazine per litre of compatible solution is recommended. Subcutaneous injection is not recommended

pH: from 4.2 to 6.2

Stability: intact ampoules can be stored at most temperatures from freezing to 40° Celsius. It should be protected from light, but a slight yellow colour does not reflect loss of potency, however a markedly discoloured solution should be discarded. Prochlorperazine does not undergo significant sorption to a 0.45 μm cellulose membrane filter during infusion

Excipients: sodium sulphite anhydrous (E221), sodium metabisulphite (E223), ethanolamine

Compatibility (Trissell 1998)

Solution compatibility: prochlorperazine is compatible with most commonly used solutions

Additive compatibility with prochlorperazine:
> **Compatible**: dexamethasone (G5W), dimenhydrinate (G5W)
> **Incompatible**: methohexitone (G5W), thiopentone

Drugs compatible with prochlorperazine in a syringe for 24 hours:
> **Compatible**: alfentanil, chlorpromazine, diamorphine, droperidol, fentanyl, hyoscine hydrobromide, metoclopramide, morphine sulphate, nalbuphine, pentazocine, pethidine, promazine, promethazine
> **Incompatible**: ketorolac, midazolam, thiopentone

Y site injection compatibility with prochlorperazine:
> **Compatible**: granisetron, heparin, hydrocortisone, ondansetron, potassium chloride, propofol
> **Incompatible**: aztreonam, tazocin

Promazine (Trissell 1998)

Presentation: promazine is available as 25 mg and 50 mg tablets, 25 mg/5 ml and 50 mg/5 ml oral solution and 50 mg/1 ml ampoule

Administration: The injection can be given by deep intramuscular injection. It can be given diluted as an intravenous injection at a concentration not exceeding 25 mg/ml. Therefore, it cannot be given undiluted. Extravasation should be avoided. It should not be given intra-arterially

pH: from 4 to 5.5

Stability: it should be stored at room temperature. It should be protected from freezing and light. A slight yellow colour does not reflect loss of potency, however a markedly discoloured solution or solutions containing precipitation should be discarded. Promazine can undergo some sorption over a number of hours through some burettes, tubing and PVC bags

Excipients: none

Compatibility (Trissell 1998)

Solution compatibility: Promazine is compatible with most commonly used solutions, but some loss can occur in sodium chloride 0.9% if exposed to light

Additive compatibility with promazine:
>   **Compatible**: heparin
>   **Incompatible**: methohexitone (G5W & NS), thiopentone (G5W)

Drugs compatible with promazine in a syringe for 24 hours:
>   **Compatible**: droperidol, fentanyl, glycopyrrolate, hyoscine hydrobromide, metoclopramide, midazolam, morphine sulphate, pentazocine, pethidine, prochlorperazine, promethazine
>   **Incompatible**: not known

Y site injection compatibility with prochlorperazine: no data

Promethazine hydrochloride (Phenergan) (Anon 1998b)

Presentation: promethazine is available as 10 mg and 25 mg tablets, 5 mg/5 ml elixir and 25 mg/1 ml and 50 mg/2 ml ampoule

Administration: the injection can be given by deep intramuscular injection. It can be given undiluted as an intravenous injection into tubing of a running infusion solution at a rate not exceeding 25 mg/min or by slow intravenous injection after diluting to 2.5 mg/ml with water for injection. It can also be given by continuous or intermittent intravenous infusion. Extravasation should be avoided. It should not be given subcutaneously or intra-arterially

pH: from 4 to 5.5

Excipients: sodium sulphite anhydrous (E211), sodium metabisulphite (E223)

Stability: it should be stored at room temperature. It should be protected from freezing and light. It has increasing stability with decreasing pH. Promethazine undergoes significant sorption through silastic sorption but not polyethylene tubing

Compatibility (Trissell 1998)

Solution compatibility: promethazine is compatible with most commonly used solutions

Additive compatibility with promethazine:
>**Compatible**: not known
>**Incompatible**: heparin, methohexitone (G5W), thiopentone

Drugs compatible with promethazine in a syringe for 24 hours:
>**Compatible**: atropine plus pethidine, chlorpromazine, droperidol, fentanyl, glycopyrrolate, hyoscine hydrobromide, metoclopramide, midazolam, morphine sulphate, nalbuphine, pentazocine, pethidine, prochlorperazine, promazine
>**Incompatible**: heparin, ketorolac, thiopentone

Y site injection compatibility with promethazine:
>**Compatible**: aztreonam, ciprofloxacin, granisetron, hydrocortisone, ondansetron, potassium chloride
>**Incompatible**: most cephalosporins, heparin, tazocin

Propofol (Diprivan) (Anon 1998b)

Propofol is an intravenous anaesthetic that has been shown to have anti-emetic properties at its best to be non-emetogenic at its worst. It is included in here for completeness.

Presentation: propofol is a ready to use oil in water emulsion in two concentrations: 1% and 2%. The 1% product is available as 20 ml ampoules, 50 ml and 100 ml vials, 50 ml prefilled syringes. The 2% product is available as a 50 ml prefilled syringe

Administration: Propofol should be well shaken before use. It is usually administered undiluted as an intravenous injection or infusion. It can also be diluted in 5% glucose to a dilution of not less than 2 mg/ml. This is not recommended as propofol is not a preserved product against antimicrobials, and many outbreaks of postoperative infection have occurred. Filters with a pore size less than 5 μm should not be used with propofol because they may restrict the administration and/or cause the breakdown of the emulsion

pH: from 7 to 8.5

Stability: unopened containers should not be kept in a refrigerator, but away from light. Propofol undergoes oxidative generation when exposed to oxygen. Any unused propofol should be discarded 12 hours after spiking the vial. Extreme caution should be taken when adding anything to propofol as it supports microbiological growth. Ideally, no additions should be made, but if any additions are made, they should be done under strict aseptic conditions

Excipients: glycerol, nitrogen, purified egg phosphatide, sodium hydroxide, soybean oil

Compatibility (Trissell 1998)

Drugs compatible with propofol in a syringe for 24 hours:

  Compatible: thiopentone

  Incompatible: not known

Y site injection compatibility with propofol:

  Compatible: alfentanil, buprenorphine, chlorpromazine, dexamethasone, droperidol, fentanyl, granisetron, haloperidol, hydromorphone, ketamine, levorphanol, lorazepam, metoclopramide, midazolam, morphine sulphate, nalbuphine, pancuronium, pethidine, sufentanil, vecuronium

  Incompatible: atracurium, cisatracurium, mivacurium

Tropisetron (Navoban) (Anon 1998b)

Presentation: 5 mg capsules and 5 mg/5 ml ampoules.
Administration: The injection can be given as a slow intravenous injection or into a running infusion or as an intravenous infusion diluted in 100 ml sodium chloride 0.9%
pH: from 5.0 to 5.1 (Georget *et al.* 1997)
Stability: tropisetron should be stored below 25 °C. Diluted solutions are stable for up to 24 hours. Diluted solutions are stable for up to three months in PVC or polyolefin bags when stored in a fridge or freezer (Georget *et al.* 1997) or in polyethylene containers or polypropylene syringes for up to two weeks (Brigas *et al.* 1998)
Excipients: not known
Compatibility
Solution compatibility: tropisetron is sodium chloride 0.9%, Ringer's solution, fructose 5% and glucose 5%

Additive compatibility with tropisetron:
        Compatible: not known
        Incompatible: not known

Drugs compatible with tropisetron in a syringe for 24 hours:
        Compatible: not known
        Incompatible: not known

Y site injection compatibility with tropisetron:
        Compatible: not known
        Incompatible: not known

References

Allcutt, D.A., Lort, D. & McCullum, C.N. (1983). Final in-line filtration for intravenous infusions: a prospective hospital study. *British Journal of Surgery* **70**, 111–13.

Anon. (1993). *The incidence and impact of post-operative nausea* (Glaxo Wellcome, Data on file). Synergy Medical Education, London.

Anon. (1998a). *Directory of operating theatres and departments of surgery.* London.

Anon. (1998b). *ABPI Compendium of data sheets and summaries of product characteristics 1998–99.* Datapharm Publications Ltd, London.

Aronson, J.K. (1995). Routes of drug administration. 5. Intramuscular injection. *Prescribers Journal* **35**, 32–36.

Backhouse, C.M., Ball, P.R., Booth, S. *et al.* (1987). Particulate contaminants of intravenous medications and infusions. *Journal of Pharmacy and Pharmacology* **39**, 241–245.

Baumgartner, T.G., Schmidt, G.L., Thakker, K.M. *et al.* (1986). Bacterial endotoxin retention by in-line filters. *American Journal of Hospital Pharmacy* **43**, 681–684.

Bradley, K. (1996). Swap data on drug compatibilities. *Pharmacy in Practice* **3**, 69–72.

Brigas, F., Sautou-Miranda, V., Normand, B. *et al.* (1998). Compatibility of tropisetron with glass and plastics. Stability under different storage conditions. *Journal of Pharmacy and Pharmacology* **50**, 407–411.

Clayton, D.G., Shanahan, E.C., Ordman, A.J. & Simpson, J.C. (1985). Contamination of the internal jugular cannulae. *Anaesthesia* **40**, 523–528.

Cousins, D.H. & Upton, D.R. (1998). Medication errors. Why we must now act in theatre. *Pharmacy in Practice* **8**, 64–66.

Dann, T.C. (1969). Routine skin preparation before injection: unnecessary procedure. *Lancet* ii, 96–98.

De Luca, P.P., Rappm R.P., Bivins, B.A. *et al.* (1976). Filtration and infusion phlebitis: a double blind prospective clinical study. *American Journal of Hospital Pharmacy* **33**, 29–34.

Dhami, S.S., Gahir, B.S., Hall, G. & Hall, S.M. (1995). *Pharmaceutical Journal* **255**(6868), R33.

Driscoll, D.F., Lewis, K. & Bistrian, B. (1997). Particle size distribution of propofol injection ampules and vials: the benefits of filtration. *International Journal of Pharmaceutical Compounding* **1**.

Falchuk, K.H., Peterson, L. & McNeil, B.J. (1985). Microparticulate-induced phlebitis: its prevention by in-line filtration. *New England Journal of Medicine* **312**, 78–82.

Francombe, P. (1998). Intravenous filters and phlebitis. *Nursing Times* **84**, 34–35.

Georget, S., Blaise, N., Perrin, A. *et al.* (1997). Stability of refrigerated and frozen solutions of tropisetron in either polyvinylchloride or polyolefin bags. *Journal of Clinical Pharmacy and Therapeutics* **22**, 257–260.

Greenblatt, D.J. & Allen, M.D. (1978). Intramuscular injection-site complications. *Journal of the American Medical Association* **240**, 542–544.

Hipwell, C.E., Mashford, M.L. & Robertson, M.B. (ed.) (1984). *Guide to parenteral administration of drugs.* ADIS Health Science Press, Sydney.

Holmes, C.J., Kundsin, R.B., Ausman, R.K. & Walter, C.W. (1980). Potential hazards associated with microbial contamination of in-line filters during intravenous therapy. *Journal of Clinical Microbiology* **12**, 725–731.

Macmillan, E.L. (1972). Sterile fluids for parenteral infusions. Letter to Secretaries of Hospital Management Committees, 18 August.

Maki, D.G., Rhame, F.S., Mackel, D.C. *et al.* (1971). Nosocomial septicaemia subsequent to contaminated intravenous fluid. Presented at the Annual Meeting of the American Society for Microbiology, Minneapolis, 5 May.

Marshall, L. & Lloyd, G. (1987). Intravenous fluid filtration. *Care of the Critically Ill* **3**, 10–17.

Ng, P.C., Herrington, R.A., Beane, C.A. *et al.* (1989). An outbreak of Acinetobacter septicaemia in a neonatal intensive care unit. *Journal of Hospital Infection* **14**, 363–368.

Quercia, R.A., Hills, S.Q., Klimek, J.J. *et al.* (1986). Bacteriological contamination of intravenous infusion delivery systems in an intensive care unit. *American Journal of Medicine* **80**, 364–368.

Sabon, R.L., Cheung, E.Y., Stommel, K.A. & Hennen, C.R. (1989). Glass particle contamination: influence of aspiration methods and ampule type. *Anesthesiology* **70**, 859–862.

Shaw, N.J. & Lyall, E.G.H. (1985). Hazards of glass ampules. *British Medical Journal* **291**, 1390.

Stewart, J.T., Warren, F.T., King, D.T., Venkateshwaran, T.G. & Fox, J.L. (1998). Stability of ondansetron hydrochloride and 12 medications in plastic syringes. *American Journal of Health-System Pharmacy* **55**, 2630–2634.

Taylor, S.A. (1982). Particulate contamination of sterile syringes and needles. *Journal of Pharmacy and Pharmacology* **34**, 493–495.

Trissell, L.A. (1998). *ASHP handbook on injectable drugs*, 10th edn. American Society of Healthcare Pharmacists.

Twum-Danso, K., Dawodu, A.H., Saleh, M.A.F. & Makiling, L.S. (1989). An outbreak of Klebsiella pneumoniae bacteraemia in five children on intravenous therapy. *Journal of Hospital Infection* **14**, 271–274.

Uchegbu & Florence (1996). Adverse drug events related to dosage forms and delivery systems. *Drug Safety* **14**(1), 39–67.

Wardle, E.N. (1986). Endotoxins and respiratory and renal failure. *Care of the Critically Ill* **2**, 54–56.

Whipple, J.K., Quebbeman, E.J., Lewis, K.S. *et al.* (1994). Identification of patient controlled analgesia overdose in hospitalised patients: a computerised method of monitoring adverse events. *Annals of Pharmacotherapy* **28**, 655–657.

PART 3

Clinical governance of PONV services

Practical organisation of preventive and treatment strategies: recommendations for a *modus operandi* for the clinical team

Andrew P. Vickers

Introduction

Post-operative nausea and vomiting (PONV) are distressing though not inevitable sequelae of anaesthesia and surgery. The reported incidence varies widely depending upon the populations and procedures studied but, overall, PONV affects about one third of the four million patients undergoing surgery under general anaesthesia in the UK per annum. They can lead to medical problems such as dehydration, pulmonary aspiration and delayed recovery and discharge. The patient's memory of PONV can be more profound than for pain and the fear of nausea and emesis such that patients may refuse analgesics to avoid their side-effects (Orkin 1992).

The aetiology of PONV is complex and multi-factorial; risk factors can be broadly classified as:

- Patient characteristics e.g. predisposition to PONV (previous history) or travel sickness, obesity and the female gender.
- Surgical factors e.g. site and duration of surgery, and urgency of procedure.
- Anaesthetic factors e.g. choice of anaesthetic agents, use of opioids.
- Post-operative factors e.g. consumption of opioids, time to oral intake, hypoxia, hypotension and early ambulation.

Managing post-operative nausea and vomiting

The management of PONV is a multi-modal process and can be considered under the following headings:

- Identifying those patients at risk of PONV.
- Use of prophylactic anti-emetics for those patients considered high risk of PONV.
- Minimising the use of triggering agents during anaesthesia.
- Accurate charting of nausea and vomiting scores.
- Appropriate prescriptions of anti-emetics
- Prompt treatment of PONV.

- Arrangements for special patient groups.
- Education programmes.
- Audit.
- Economics.

Identifying those patients at risk of PONV

There are many predisposing factors for PONV so priorities should be established to identify those patients most likely to experience it; for example, women with a past history of PONV undergoing major gynaecological surgery should be considered very high risk while elderly patients having cataract surgery are low risk. This assessment is important in assuring that those patients at high risk receive prophylactic measures while satisfying financial constraints and minimising side effects from anti-emetics.

Use of prophylactic anti-emetics and other techniques

Rowbotham (1992) has reviewed randomised-controlled trials (RCTs) of prophylactic anti-emetics and concluded that cyclizine, droperidol, prochlorperazine and ondansetron have a prophylactic effect while the use of metoclopramide is questionable. There are a number of issues that remain unclear, however, such as the optimum dose and ideal time of administration for all of these drugs.

A systematic review of RCTs by Vickers (1996) has demonstrated that acupuncture/acupressure administered before surgery has a prophylactic effect but not if stimulation is performed only during anaesthesia. The use of the P6 point was common to all the studies reviewed. Vickers did comment, however, that the design of all these studies was not ideal and did question his conclusion regarding the efficacy of acupuncture.

Zingiber officinale (ginger) has been shown to have anti-emetic properties; in a study of women undergoing day case laparoscopy it was as effective as metoclopramide and superior to placebo in preventing PONV (Phillips 1993).

It is important, however, to remember that *none* of these drugs/methods are totally efficacious. The dopamine-2 antagonists and anti-histamines/anti-cholinergics can have significant side-effects and 5-HT$_3$ antagonists are relatively expensive so a cost:benefit assessment is an important part of the prophylactic use of medications.

Minimising triggering agents during anaesthesia

There is conflicting evidence from two systematic reviews (Divatia *et al* 1996; Tramer *et al* 1996) whether the omission of nitrous oxide influences the incidence of PONV. All volatile agents are ematogenic whereas propofol may have significant anti-emetic properties (Watcha *et al.* 1992).

The use of local anaesthetic techniques will reduce opioid requirements both during and after surgery and would be expected to reduce the likelihood of PONV.

The selective use of nasogastric tubes during/after intra-abdominal surgery as opposed to indiscriminate gastric drainage will help to minimise PONV (Cheatham *et al.* 1995).

Charting of nausea and vomiting scores

Scores for PONV are helpful in highlighting problems and to facilitate audit. The act of recording scores helps focus attention on PONV and, when combined with guidelines for management, will encourage prompt treatment of nausea and/or vomiting. There is no universal system for assessing PONV with most departments in the UK using variations on simple numerical scales. High scores should trigger agreed procedures for managing PONV.

Appropriate prescriptions of anti-emetics

Anti-emetics fall into three broad groups, the dopamine-2 antagonists, the muscarinic antagonists and the 5-HT$_3$ antagonists. Prescriptions for these groups should take into account not only appropriate dose and dosing interval but avoid using two drugs from the same group; if one failed it is likely that another will do likewise. This is particularly important for the dopamine-2 antagonists where involuntary movement syndromes, such as oculogyric crisis and acute dystonia can be very distressing consequences of overdose.

Prompt treatment of PONV

It is most important that PONV is recognised and treated promptly. This can only happen if other factors in the process are carried out such as charting PONV scores and prescribing anti-emetics. The use of guidelines may be helpful to ensure this and should necessitate that anti-emetics are used logically for maximum effect and to minimise side effects. Established PONV should be regarded as a significant complication of surgery and medical and nursing staff should be educated to treat it as such. Failure to institute treatment early can result in other medical complications, patient distress and influence patients' attitudes to future surgery.

Arrangements for special groups

Day cases

PONV is a significant factor in unexpected overnight stay for day case patients but many patients experience PONV only after they have left the hospital. An audit of children undergoing day case dental extraction in Lancaster demonstrated that more than 25% vomited after leaving hospital. An additional factor in this may be having to endure transport home, which can last up to 60 minutes. The prescription of anti-emetics is complicated by the fact that the patient is not under supervision by medical and nursing staff and side effects may be significant. There are no systematic reviews to indicate which medication is best (efficacy versus side effects) and the optimal dose of any anti-emetic. Policies should exist for the management of PONV before discharge. Written information included with the drugs may optimise the use of medication.

Children

The incidence of PONV is relatively high in children but it is important to distinguish between emesis which does not significantly disturb the child and severe nausea and/or repeating vomiting which distresses the child and may cause biochemical disturbances. Ondansetron is licensed for the prevention and treatment of PONV in children over 2 years whereas granisetron is not recommended for this purpose (British National Formulary 2001). The use of metoclopramide for patients less than 20 years old should be restricted to severe, intractable vomiting and prochlorperazine should only be used in tablet form. Cyclizine tablets are licensed for children over 6 years of age but the injection is not (CeNeS Pharmaceuticals 2002). Guidelines would optimise PONV management.

The elderly

Prolonged pharmacokinetics may increase the risks of Parkinsonian side effects from dopamine-2 antagonists. The anti-cholinergic effects of cyclizine and hyoscine may exacerbate confusion and dementia in the elderly.

The pregnant patient

Surgery for non-delivery purposes is unusual in pregnant women. The use of any drug raises fears of teratogenicity in the first trimester and threats to foetal viability later in the pregnancy. Ondansetron, granisetron and metoclopramide have cautions for the use in pregnant patients (British National Formulary 2001) and, in the absence of definitive human data, the manufacturers do not recommend cyclizine for this purpose (CeNeS Pharmaceuticals 2002). Anti-emetics have been ranked in terms of level of risk the drug poses to the foetus (Briggs *et al.* 1994) with ondansetron, cyclizine and metoclopramide rated as 'B_m' and prochlorperazine as 'C' (see Appendix B for an explanation of these terms).

Education

Implementation of the process described above is dependent on all the carers involved in the process being aware of PONV and its management. The groups that should be targeted include anaesthetists, non-anaesthetist medical staff and nursing staff. It is unrealistic to assume that knowledge gained at, say, medical school is sufficient and contemporary for this purpose. A regular programme of education should be in place, attendance should be compulsory and written records of attendance kept. Guidelines are particularly appropriate for managing a problem that is routine but is managed by different people in different wards and departments (The Royal College of Anaesthetists and The Association of Anaesthetists 1998). They should support educational programmes to ensure best practice.

Audit

Audit is a valuable tool to examine whether local management of PONV is satisfactory. The incidence of PONV in various patient groups is well established so audit should not be continuous but target specific groups regularly for a fixed period of, say, one week. Appropriate indicators could be the incidence of PONV in that group, the percentage of patients who were prescribed an anti-emetic and the percentage of patients with PONV who received one (The Royal College of Anaesthetists 1999).

The Welsh Office (1992) has set standards for PONV with an initial target of no more than 25% of all surgical patients to suffer PONV. There was an expectation that this would fall to less than 10% but different standards would have to be set for specific groups such as major gynaecological surgery.

Economics

Post-operative nausea and vomiting can be very distressing but also have an economic impact; they may prolong hospital stay and the cost of treating each emetic episode has been calculated to be approximately £1. Against this must be balanced the use of expensive anti-emetics; the indiscriminate use of these drugs may result in restriction of their use. Once again, the use of guidelines may help to ensure that valuable resources are targeted on those most at risk of PONV (Tang *et al.* 1996).

PONV management: current practices

The factors involved in the optimal management of PONV have been described above but does how closely does actual practice match the ideal situation? Is PONV a problem? A review of textbooks will produce a list of options for management but does not describe what is actually done. To try to understand current practice for the management of PONV and why it might fail, a survey was carried out in October/November 1998 of members of the Acute Pain Special Interest Group of the Pain Society (APSIG). Two hundred and fourteen questionnaires were distributed and 131 were returned and analysed. In January 2002 a second, smaller survey of 17 members of APSIG was carried out to try to assess if there had been any changes in practise in the past three years. In considering the results of these surveys it must be understood that:

* This is a self-selected group; it is reasonable to assume that anaesthetists or nurses who are motivated to be members of APSIG and the Pain Society are enthusiastic about pain and PONV management and represent the better end of the spectrum of practice.
* It is possible that in the 1998 survey more than one member of a department is a member of APSIG and so multiple entries from a single department have been received; it is the author's opinion that this will not significantly affect the outcome of the survey.

• Where the 2002 survey revisited areas explored in the 1998 survey, the results of the later study are recorded in italics adjacent to the 1998 results.

Have you audited PONV in your hospital?
     n = 131   Yes   94 (72%)   No   37 (28%)

Have you audited PONV in your hospital in 2001?
      2002   Yes   37%   No   63%

The responses to this question indicate that some audit has been carried out in many of the departments sampled but does not define how recently this was done, whether audit is recurrent or which groups of patients were targeted.

Do you know the incidence of PONV in your hospital?
     n = 131   Yes   67 (51%)   No   64 (49%)
     2002   *31%*   *69%*

Some responses gave an indication of the actual figures for incidence of PONV but this was not specifically sought since the incidence varies so widely between different patient groups.

Do you provide teaching on PONV management to:
New anaesthetists?	Yes	81 (62%)	No	42 (32%)
2002		*75%*		*25%*
Other new doctors?	Yes	51 (39%)	No	78 (60%)
2002		*67%*		*33%*
Nursing staff?	Yes	85 (65%)	No	44 (34%)
2002		*94%*		*6%*

Education for all these groups is the cornerstone to the management of PONV. The responses to this question indicate that some educational activity is being done but, bearing in mind that the population sampled for this survey represents the better end of the spectrum, these results are disappointing. The results from 2002 suggest an overall improvement in the situation. In general terms, the departments which were providing education were also the ones who had guidelines for the management of PONV in place (vide infra).

All three groups who received training are important links in the chain for providing optimal management of PONV in terms of prophylactic anti-emetics, avoiding triggers and prescribing anti-emetics (anaesthetists), supervising treatment and modifying medication (ward doctors), and charting observations and treating PONV (nurses). Ensuring that they understand their responsibilities must be a priority.

Do you have guidelines/policies (circle whichever appropriate) for the use of anti-emetics in the following situations:

Recovery?	Yes	70 (53%)	No	60 (46%)
Inpatient prophylaxis?	Yes	53 (40%)	No	77 (60%)
2002		*63%*		*37%*
Inpatient treatment?	Yes	70 (53%)	No	57 (44%)
2002		*81%*		*19%*
Day case prophylaxis?	Yes	49 (37%)	No	78 (60%)
Day case take home/	Yes	30 (23%)	No	94 (72%)
2002		*53%*		*47%*
Paediatric prophylaxis/	Yes	27 (21%)	No	84 (64%)
Paediatric treatment?	Yes	41 (31%)	No	77 (59%)
2002		*47%*		*53%*
Paediatric take home/	Yes	7 (5%)	No	96 (73%)

Some questionnaires had blank responses for one or more of these categories which accounts for missing percentages. Where a preference was expressed for guidelines or protocols (6 responses), this was always for guidelines.

Guidelines can play a major part in the training of staff. They have an invaluable role in some situations such as managing rare or life-threatening events but are very useful also in providing a co-ordinated response to a problem that spans a number of different clinical areas and different groups of staff such as PONV. Guidelines should not automatically be regarded as limiting clinical freedom but encouraging best practice and should be modified in the light of developing information and experience (The Royal College of Anaesthetists and The Association of Anaesthetists 1998). Unfortunately, the 1998 survey has shown that departments that do not provide comprehensive education programmes do not have guidelines in place either. An example of a guideline for adult PONV can be found in Appendix A.

*In your hospital, which of the following drugs are used regularly for (includes multiple responses): Note figures represent **percentage** of total respondents with figures in parentheses indicating the 2002 survey.*

	Prochlorperazine	Metoclopramide	Droperidol	Cyclizine	Ondansetron
Prophylaxis	27 (19)	47 (13)	56 (0)	42 (56)	59 (69)
Treatment	79 (75)	63 (25)	34 (0)	77 (94)	71 (88)
Paediatrics	17 (0)	23 (0)	8 (0)	27 (38)	40 (88)
Day case TTO	1 (0)	15 (6)	3 (0)	6 (6)	6 (6)

Dexamethasone is used in 2 departments for prophylaxis and 1 for treatment, domperidone is used in 5 and 4 respectively and in 2 departments for children.

Multiple anti-emetics are used in some departments, the most common combinations being cyclizine/ondansetron (11 responses), cyclizine/prochlorperazine (5), cyclizine/droperidol (4) and ondansetron/droperidol (3).

There is wide variation in the drugs used with most departments employing a variety of different agents. There are some published comparative studies of anti-emetics (Gan *et al.* 1994; Alexander & Fenelly 1997; Fujii *et al.* 1997) which suggest that the 5-HT$_3$ antagonists ondansetron and granisetron are superior to droperidol and metoclopramide. Tramer *et al.* (1997), however, in a systematic review of ondansetron in the treatment of *established* PONV failed to show any significant difference between ondansetron, droperidol and metoclopramide. Overall, then, there seems to be insufficient evidence to recommend any particular drug. The use of metoclopramide for prophylaxis is debatable (Rowbotham 1992) as is its use in children in view of the increased risks of involuntary movements such as akathesia. There has been a significant reduction in the use of this drug between 1998 and 2002. Choice of agents, therefore, should be based on side-effect profile and cost. The 5-HT$_3$ antagonists have an excellent side-effects profile but are considerably more expensive than either the dopamine-2 antagonists or the anti-muscarinics. These costs must be weighed against the suffering and the economic costs of PONV. Granisetron is used in some departments but not as widely as the more established ondansetron; the former has a longer duration of action. The advantages of using an agent with a long duration and minimal side effects, and avoiding the need for repeat administration may assist decision making.

There is very little evidence to guide the use of anti-emetic combinations although Puejo *et al.* (1996) did show in 100 patients that the combination of droperidol 2.5 mg and ondansetron 4 mg was more effective than either drug alone. The same drugs mixed with morphine in PCA produced a significant reduction in nausea in the first 12 hours after major gynaecological surgery compared with each individual agent (Wrench *et al.* 1996).

Do you regularly mix anti-emetics with analgesics in PCA syringes? If so, which drugs do you commonly use? n = 131

Yes	62 (47%)	No	55 (42%)
2002	*13%*		*83%*

Droperidol	51
Cyclizine	14
Ondansetron	5
Granisetron	1
Haloperidol	1
Cyclizine/ondansetron	1

There are published data to support the use of anti-emetics in the PCA syringe on efficacy grounds. For example, droperidol 0.166 mg/ml added to morphine significantly reduces emetic episodes compared to morphine alone but at the cost of increased sedation (Russell *et al.* 1996). The withdrawal of droperidol probably accounts for the major reduction in the use of opioid/anti-emetic combinations in PCA. Metoclopramide 0.5mg/ml mixed with morphine was compared with morphine alone by PCA (Walder & Aitkenhead 1994). The mixture reduced the incidence of moderate to severe nausea but not the overall incidence of nausea.

The addition of anti-emetics to morphine in PCA syringes has a tempting logic; every time the patient receives the triggering agent (morphine) he also receives the 'antidote'. There are some important issues here, though, concerning drug stability, asepsis (especially when many departments buy in sterile preparations of pre-diluted morphine) and the fact that those patients who will not experience distressing PONV must also receive drugs with not insignificant side effects.

Do you use other techniques for managing PONV?

Acupuncture/acupressure	14
Sea Bands	7
Scopaderm (no longer in BNF)	3
Buccastem (prochlorperazine)	2
Reflexology	2
Haloperidol	1
Ginger	1
Inhaled 'Mediswab'	1

The use of acupuncture has been validated but only if it is applied before induction of anaesthesia. It is assumed that Sea Bands have a similar mechanism of action as acupuncture.

In your hospital do you think PONV is well managed/a problem/no idea?

The questionnaire had two visual analogue scales relating to inpatients and day cases respectively. One end of each scale was labelled 'well managed' and the other 'a problem'; a final option was a tick box labelled 'no idea'. There is no intention to submit these results to statistical analysis so, in order to make results clearer, the visual analogue scales were divided into three equal sections that were recorded as 'well managed', 'a problem' and 'a major problem'. The responses to the inpatient question were also assessed in respect of whether the respondent had carried out audit of PONV or not.

	Well managed	A problem	A major problem	No idea
Inpatient	39 (30%)	46 (36%)	37 (29%)	7 (5%)
% who had audited	90%	67%	62%	
2002	20%	80%		
Day case	45 (35%)	32 (25%)	19 (15%)	31 (25%)
2002	58%	25%		17%

There are grounds for optimism here with 30% of respondents feeling that inpatient PONV is well managed and most of these opinions are founded on the basis of audit. In addition one third felt that PONV in day cases is managed well. However, if we bear in mind that this survey reflects the practices and results of well-motivated specialists, there is still room for considerable improvement. Nearly two thirds of respondents felt that PONV was still a problem in their hospital and the majority had audit evidence for this. The small number of 'no idea' responses for inpatients suggests that most contributors are well aware of the problem of PONV in their hospitals. The 2002 results suggest there is still a long way to go despite the efforts of medical and nursing staff.

The situation for day cases is less clear with 25% of those questioned having no idea about the incidence of PONV. Audit of day case patients is more difficult than for inpatients. Postal questionnaires may have a poor response rate and may be biased to those subjects whose experiences have been unpleasant. Telephone follow up generates a better response rate and should minimise bias but is time consuming. Despite these reservations, however, one third of respondents felt that PONV is well managed for day cases and this is a positive finding.

Conclusions

Post-operative nausea and vomiting can cause patient distress, medical complications and has financial implications. The aetiology of PONV is multi-factorial and management is a multi-modal process.

A logical approach to the management of PONV is hindered by a deficiency of systematic reviews of anti-emetics in terms of optimal dose, dosing intervals, time of administration for prophylaxis and combinations of drugs. Until these are available, management should be based on side effects and economics with a treatment pathway based on local guidelines.

The practical value of alternative techniques such as acupuncture is unclear.

Teaching the management of PONV should be a priority. It should begin before doctors and nurses have responsibility for patient care and continue throughout their careers. The provision of education programmes in the workplace is time consuming and must be repeated at regular intervals. It is unrealistic to expect training to be done in spare time, employers should provide recognised time for this both for trainers and trainees. The employment of a specialist nurse in pain and PONV management is an important contribution to this process.

Guidelines should be introduced to encourage best practice. National guidelines should be produced which can be adapted for local use.

Audit should be used to identify problem areas and to assess progress within the local service.

The effective management of PONV remains a problem in many hospitals despite efforts to improve matters.

References

Alexander, R. & Fenelly, M. (1997). Comparison of ondansetron, metoclopramide and placebo as premedicants to reduce nausea and vomiting after major surgery. *Anaesthesia* **52**, 695–698.

Briggs, G., Freeman, R. & Yaffe, S. (1994). In *Drugs in pregnancy and lactation: a reference guide to fetal and neonatal risk*, 4th edition. Williams & Wilkins: Baltimore, USA.

British Medical Journal and Royal Pharmaceutical Society of Great Britain (2001). *British National Formulary*. Royal Pharmaceutical Society of Great Britain, London.

CeNeS Pharmaceuticals (2002). *Valoid (cyclizine) monograph*. CeNeS Pharmaceuticals, Basingstoke, Hampshire, UK.

Cheatham, M., Chapman, W., Key, S. & Sawyers, J. (1995). A meta-analysis of selective versus routine nasogastric decompression after elective laparotomy. *Annals of Surgery* **221**, 469–478.

Divatia, J., Vaidya, J., Badwe, R. & Hawaldar, R. (1996). Omission of nitrous oxide during anaesthesia reduces the incidence of postoperative nausea and vomiting – a meta-analysis. *Anesthesiology* **85**, 1055–1062.

Fujii, Y., Toyooka, H. & Tanaka, H. (1997). Prevention of postoperative nausea and vomiting with granisetron, droperidol and metoclopramide in female patients with a history of motion sickness. *Canadian Journal of Anaesthesia* **44**, 820–824.

Gan, T., Collis, R. & Hetreed, M. (1994). Double-blind comparison of ondansetron, droperidol and saline in the prevention of postoperative nausea and vomiting. *British Journal of Anaesthesia*, **72**, 544–547.

Orkin, F. (1992). What do patients want? Preferences for immediate postoperative recovery. *Anaesthesia and Analgesia* **74**, 5225.

Phillips, S., Ruggier, R. & Hutchinson, S. (1993). *Zingiber officinale* (ginger) – an antiemetic for day case surgery. *Anaesthesia* **48**, 715–717.

Pueyo, F., Carrascosa, F., Lopez, L., Iribarrau, M., Garcia Pedrajas, F. & Saez, A. (1996). Combination of ondansetron and droperidol in the prophylaxis of postoperative nausea and vomiting. *Anesthesia and Analgesia* **83**(1), 117–122.

Rowbotham, D. (1992). Current management of postoperative nausea and vomiting. *British Journal of Anaesthesia* **69** (Suppl. 1), S46–S59.

The Royal College of Anaesthetists and The Association of Anaesthetists (1998). *Good Practice – a Guide for Departments of Anaesthesia*. Royal College of Anaesthetists, London.

The Royal College of Anaesthetists (1999). *Raising the Standard*. Royal College of Anaesthetists, London.

Russell, D., Duncan, L., Frame, W., Higgins, S., Asbury, A. & Millar, K. (1996). Patient controlled analgesia with morphine and droperidol following caesarian section under spinal anaesthesia. *Acta Anaesthesiologica Scandinavica* **40**, 600–605.

Tang, J., Watcha, M. & White, P. (1996). A comparison of costs and efficacy of ondansetron and droperidol as prophylactic antiemetic treatment for elective gynaecological surgery. *Anesthesia and Analgesia* **83**, 304–313.

Tramer, M., Moore, A. & McQuay, H. (1996). Omitting nitrous oxide in general anaesthesia: meta-analysis of intraoperative awareness and postoperative emesis in randomized controlled trials. *British Journal of Anaesthesia* **76**, 186–193.

Tramer, M., Moore, A., Reynolds, D. & McQuay, H. (1997). A qualitative systematic review of ondansetron in the treatment of established postoperative nausea and vomiting. *British Medical Journal* **314**, 1088–1092.

Vickers, A. (1996). Can acupuncture have specific effects on health?: a systematic review of acupuncture antiemesis trials. *Journal of the Royal Society of Medicine* **89**, 303–311.

Walder, A. & Aitkenhead, A. (1994). Antiemetic efficacy of metoclopramide when included in a patient-controlled analgesia infusion. *Anaesthesia* **49**, 804–806.

Watcha, M. & White, P. (1992). Postoperative nausea and vomiting – its etiology, treatment and prevention. *Anesthesiology* **77**, 162–184.

The Welsh Office (1992). Welsh Health Planning Forum.

Wrench, I., Ward, J., Walder, A. & Hobbs, G. (1996). The prevention of postoperative nausea and vomiting using a combination of ondansetron and droperidol. *Anaesthesia* **51**, 776–778.

Appendix A

Guideline and algorithm for managing adult PONV

■ PONV can cause dehydration and electrolyte imbalance, disrupt surgical wounds, and slow recovery.
■ PONV can have many causes, all of which are additive. Try to minimise pain, ensure rest and adequate hydration. Encourage patients to inform staff at an early stage if they feel unwell.
■ Try to identify those at most risk of PONV and treat prophylactically for the first 24 hours post-op.
  – e.g. one drug regularly and another PRN from a different class of drug.
■ Anti-emetic drugs are not always effective and may need to be given in combination with $H_1 + D_2$ antagonists such as cyclizine and prochlorperazine.
■ Check the PONV score from the PCA epidural or observation charts, assess 4 hourly or more frequently if indicated.

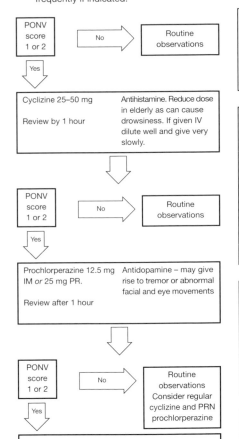

PONV Assessment Score

0 = no nausea or vomiting
1 = nausea or vomiting x 1
2 = severe nausea and vomiting > 1
X = anti-emetic given

Risk Factors

- Emergency surgery
- Major abdominal surgery
- Gynaecology, ENT and eye surgery
- Previous history of PONV
- Post-operative ileus
- Obesity
- Women more so than men
- History of travel sickness
- Anxiety and distress
- Planned early mobilisation
- Low blood pressure

Other anti-emetic therapies

- Ondansetron 5-HT_3 inhibitor, used mainly for nausea associated with chemotherapy. May cause headache or flushing.
- Metoclopramide dopamine and 5-HT_3 antagonist. Least effective anti-emetic (no better than placebo in some trials) but can relieve full feeling in stomach. Not to be used after upper GI or gastric surgery.

Management of anti-emetic side-effects

- Extrapyramidal effects such as tremor, dystonia – particularly of the head and neck and abnormal eye movements – can be reversed by giving 1–2 mg of Benztropine given IM or IV (0.5–1 mg in the elderly)

Appendix B

Risk factors for foetal harm (from Briggs *et al.* 1994).

Category A

Controlled studies in women fail to demonstrate a risk to the foetus in the first trimester (and there is no evidence of a risk in later trimesters) and the possibility of foetal harm seems remote.

Category B

Either animal-reproduction studies have not demonstrated a foetal risk but there are no controlled studies in pregnant women or animal-reproduction studies have shown an adverse effect (other than a decrease in fertility) that was not confirmed in controlled studies in women in the first trimester (and there is no evidence of a risk in later trimesters).

Category C

Either studies in animals have revealed adverse effects on the foetus (teratogenic or embryocidal or other) and there are no controlled studies in women or studies in women and animals are not available. Drugs should be given only if the potential benefit justifies the potential risk to the foetus.

Subscript 'm' e.g. B_m

Indicates that the manufacturer has rated its product in its professional literature.

Acknowledgements

The author thanks Dr David Counsell for permission to publish his algorithm for managing PONV.

Chapter 8

Clinical practice guidelines and systems of audit for the prevention and management of post-operative nausea and vomiting

Greg Hobbs, Roger Knaggs and Trudy Towell

Introduction

The multifactorial aetiology of post-operative nausea and vomiting (PONV) has often been used to explain the failure of (single) drug therapy in reducing the incidence of PONV. This is supported by increasing evidence from research practice suggesting significant reductions in PONV incidence after the use of combination anti-emetic prophylaxis. However, contemporaneous audits are likely to demonstrate that outcomes from PONV remain unacceptable in most institutions; for many patient groups, PONV incidence will be noticeably higher than those associated with published research. The challenge for those in clinical practice is to reduce this 'PONV gap' by introducing a local policy for managing PONV. Such a policy should address the inevitable delay in getting research evidence into local clinical practice. This challenge should not be underestimated. This chapter discusses the evidence and other relevant information for developing and implementing a local policy for improving PONV outcomes. A template is suggested for such a policy, upon which local considerations and priorities can be developed. The key contributions of a multidisciplinary approach, clinical guidelines and audit are highlighted.

Developing and implementing a new policy
What are the barriers to improving outcomes?

Getting research evidence into clinical practice and the organisation of PONV management are the fundamental problems.

PONV incidence in clinical practice is noticeably higher than in published randomised, controlled trials. The barriers to successful application of research evidence to health care include the size and complexity of the research, difficulties in developing evidence-based clinical policy and practical problems such as lack of access to guidelines, organisational barriers, ineffectual education programmes and low staff adherence to recommendations (Haynes *et al.* 1998). Several general steps have been suggested to overcome potential barriers (NHS Centre for Reviews and Dissemination 1999).

The management of PONV has two main components; prevention and treatment. These may be disparate and fragmented in clinical practice. For example, although anaesthetists have specialist knowledge and skills highly relevant to both components, for the most part, prevention has largely been the domain of the anaesthetist. During their pre-operative patient assessment, the anaesthetist usually makes a judgement of PONV risk and may give single, and increasingly combination anti-emetic prophylaxis during surgery if the patient is considered to be 'at risk'. The prescription for later treatment of PONV is usually made by an anaesthetist based in operating theatres.

There are several problems with this approach. The importance given to the risk assessment and subsequent clinical actions is likely to vary according to other clinical priorities. There is little evidence of the accuracy of this informal risk assessment and if subsequent actions taken by the anaesthetist are appropriate for that risk. Later treatment of established PONV in the ward environment is done by nursing staff and not the anaesthetist. This fragments the PONV management pathway and may reduce ownership of clinical responsibility for patient outcomes.

The management of PONV also lacks glamour. PONV is neither a critical incident nor major morbidity and rarely causes death. There are no national targets or political imperatives (although the Welsh Office has previously made some initiatives). Without a reputation for 'seriousness', PONV attracts scant interest from professionals who control the resources available for peri-operative care. Other than existing expenditure on anti-emetic drugs and relevant disposables, there are no specific resources or budget dedicated to the management of PONV.

Inadequate or inappropriate knowledge, attitudes and expectations of patients and staff alike do not facilitate change. Acute pain service personnel have been able to demonstrate improvements in these variables with appropriate education; this should also be possible in PONV management. It is also unlikely that all professionals and patients will be aware of their roles and responsibilities in the process of managing PONV without intensive and ongoing education and training both inside and outside the theatre environment. Few institutions will have explicit goals or standards for outcomes from PONV management. A lack of effective leadership must also be a major factor contributing to poor outcomes. Who has formal accountability for basic humanitarian outcomes such as PONV in your institution?

What are appropriate implementation strategies?

One of the key aims of a PONV management policy is to promote uptake of evidence into clinical practice. A new policy is more likely to be successful if certain 'preconditions' and the evidence about the effectiveness of various implementation strategies are considered before implementation.

Preconditions that may influence the uptake of new evidence (Rubin *et al.* 2000) include:

- Availability of good information or evidence
- Ready access to this evidence
- An environment that supports and encourages use of the best evidence
- Effective mechanisms for promoting knowledge uptake

The initial assembly of the evidence for PONV management has been ably assisted by systematic reviews and sources of information such as this book. However, to be both evidence based and clinically useful, policy must balance the strengths and weaknesses of relevant research with the realities of the clinical setting (Gray *et al.* 1997). A range of non-evidence based factors including historical and cultural influences will inevitably mould policy and its effectiveness; policy must be adapted to local circumstances (Haynes *et al.* 1998).

For example, the mechanisms chosen for local promotion of knowledge uptake may be crucial. Reliance on traditional continuing education alone to change performance will disappoint (Davis *et al.* 1995). Education in PONV management has been identified previously as needing improvement (Wilder-Smith *et al.* 1997). Experience in PONV service development suggests that multidisciplinary education, including patients and professionals, is essential for improving outcomes. This may be more effective if it occurs within a supportive, local clinical environment, is highly interactive and makes patient and staff roles and responsibilities clear before the event. A range of interventions and implementation strategies can be applied locally. These have been evaluated in systematic reviews (Bero *et al.* 1998; NHS Centre for Reviews and Dissemination 1999; Grol *et al.* 1999). Table 8.1 outlines these interventions and their effectiveness. Most of these interventions are applicable to PONV management. Awareness of this evidence is likely to enhance policy effectiveness if it is incorporated into policy development and implementation. For example, those who view guidelines (alone) as an ineffective change instrument are probably right. The key message is that policy must use a combination of interventions, such as local consensus meetings and patient involvement in formulating policy, as well as interactive education, audit and feedback and decision support systems e.g. algorithms, guidelines and sticky label reminders.

Why a multidisciplinary policy for PONV management?

Viewed simplistically, it is easy to assume that PONV is merely a temporary inconvenience for the patient and for the staff directly involved in managing the problem, notably recovery room and ward nursing staff. More extensive analysis reveals PONV to be complex and multifactorial, influenced by considerations including pre-operative patient preparation, individual patient risk factors, intra-operative interventions and post-operative management techniques. It is therefore not surprising that PONV in adults has remained at a consistent rate of between 20% and 30% (Adriani *et al.* 1961; Cohen *et al.* 1994) and that dependence on post-operative

Table 8.1 Implementation strategies and their effectiveness (from Rubin *et al.* 2000)

Consistently effective*
Educational outreach visits
Interactive educational meetings
Decision support systems (e.g. stickers, reminders)
Multifaceted interventions (combining audit & feedback, reminders, local consensus
processes, marketing)
Mass media interventions

Variable effectiveness*
Audit and feedback
Local consensus processes
Patient-mediated interventions (patient involvement)

Little or no effect
Educational materials (e.g. clinical guidelines alone, audiovisual or electronic materials)
Didactic educational meetings

Unknown effectiveness
Financial incentives, administrative interventions (regulations, laws)

* Most interventions can be applied to PONV management.

intervention by recovery room and ward nursing staff has failed to reduce this level of incidence.

Further reductions in the incidence of PONV can only be achieved by improved pharmacological prophylaxis, less emetogenic anaesthetic techniques, better pain and anti-emesis management and less invasive surgical technique (Tramér 2001). This is dependent on the implementation of a range of measures by various members of the multidisciplinary team and will only be achieved if personnel are aware of the problem, have the necessary resources available to them and the knowledge and application to select and apply them appropriately. It is therefore evident that both the organisation and clinical process for managing PONV require changing. Sustained, local improvement in outcomes from PONV needs widespread, permanent changes to clinical practice both in the traditional anaesthetic and theatre environment as well as hospital wards. An effective strategy for improving outcomes from PONV must examine pre-operative, intra-operative and post-operative care relevant to the management of PONV. This can only be effective if it is multidisciplinary.

Team working may be a key factor in the effectiveness of new clinical policy (McNicol *et al.* 1993). Such models for introducing clinical guidelines and reducing inconsistencies in practice are available. The acute pain service (APS) and the integrated care pathway are examples (Campbell *et al.* 1998). 'The Anaesthesia Team' (Association of Anaesthetists of Great Britain and Ireland 1998) promotes the concept of multidisciplinary working in peri-operative care.

Multidisciplinary anti-emesis teams?

Described as the 'big little problem' (Fisher 1997), PONV holds a position of low significance in the overall scheme of surgical management and as such is unlikely to attract specific funding to enable the establishment of a team with the definitive remit of reducing PONV. This is neither necessary nor sufficient.

More than half the hospitals in the UK have established acute pain teams (Audit Commission 1997). Other hospitals have adopted alternative approaches to deal with the multidisciplinary issue of pain management by initiating pain management groups or devolving responsibility for change to a designated existing group. Providing such groups have multiprofessional representation there is no reason to create a further specialist team.

The role of the Acute Pain Service

PONV and post-operative pain have a striking number of similarities. Their occurrence is common and unpleasant. They are multifactorial in nature and have implications for post-operative morbidity and prolongation of hospital stay. They can both be improved by changing peri-operative management strategies. Drug therapy is a current keystone to their management. Finally, successful amelioration is dependent upon engaging a large number of health care workers from a range of professions in the adoption and maintenance of changes to their normal practice.

However, it is impractical to assume that specialist nurses within an APS can take direct responsibility for the management of PONV; at our institution this would necessitate visits to more than 40,000 patients each year. Neither is this approach desirable. One of the criticisms frequently levelled at specialist nurses is that they de-skill nursing colleagues by taking over specific elements of care (Humphris 1994). As with pain management our approach is to increase the skills of colleagues, giving them the knowledge, authority, confidence and support to function autonomously within the multidisciplinary team, an issue that is critical in terms of changing practice and improving patient outcomes (Fulton 1997). The APS therefore has important leadership, training and supportive roles.

Key members of the multidisciplinary team

In addition to specialist APS nurses, other clinical staff can strongly influence outcomes from PONV management. These roles must be considered when developing PONV policy.

The anaesthetic contribution

Identification of an individual with responsibility for the quality of PONV management is an important part of policy. For obvious reasons, anaesthetists are usually best placed to lead the development of multidisciplinary vehicles for improving outcomes in PONV management. Established clinical and managerial roles should be exploited, particularly those working in acute pain services. Formalising a lead responsibility and accountability for PONV outcomes (even better with dedicated time, surely a rare achievement) will help raise the profile and impetus for change. However, each individual anaesthetist can have a profound effect on PONV outcomes during a relatively short period of the patient's hospital stay. It is therefore each clinician's responsibility to adopt evidence-based practices and techniques that optimise PONV outcomes, and to disseminate best practice within their department.

The pharmacy contribution

Drug therapy has become the mainstay of modern PONV management. Hospital pharmacists have extensive knowledge and access to clinical and economic information about drugs as well as experience of enhancing effective drug use in hospitals. Improving outcomes from the management of PONV will usually include a change in drug practice. Pharmacists have other relevant skills and regular professional contact with all types of staff as well as patients in the ward environment. Pharmacists are therefore well suited to contribute to a multidisciplinary PONV management framework including roles in education, guideline development and implementation, continuous clinical and economic monitoring, and research. This may make some additional demands on pharmacist time. Historically, hospital pharmacists were employed mainly in the manufacture and supply of medicines. Largely these activities have now been delegated to more appropriately qualified technical staff, thus releasing time for pharmacists to be more involved with the promotion of safe, effective and economic use of medicines, particularly at ward and department level.

A ready source for medicines information

The published literature contains an overwhelming amount of research data on anti-emetic drugs. This grows by the month. Both quality and applicability to current practice need to be assessed and critical appraisal is essential to ensure that decision-making about drug use is based on objective evidence. It is neither practical nor a good use of time for most clinicians to be regularly reviewing this literature in detail. Drug information pharmacists, located in most hospitals, have ready access to a variety of medical, pharmacy and nursing databases and are experienced in reviewing the literature on a regular basis. With ready access to such information, pharmacists are well placed to collate and maintain the evidence for clinical guideline development. In addition, pharmacists may use these skills to assess and decide the place of new drugs in routine clinical practice.

Implementing change in drug use

Developing and implementing guidelines for the use of drugs by medical and nursing staff is never straightforward. In addition to education of different groups of staff, there are several organisational hurdles that must be overcome. Other groups invariably become involved when changes to drug utilisation are expected, particularly when an additional cost is anticipated. Such groups might include drug and therapeutics committees who oversee the use of drugs within hospitals, budget holders who must pay the bill, and risk management committees. Many pharmacists have developed skills in pharmaco-economic evaluation that are relevant to this area. Pharmacists are therefore well placed to co-ordinate guideline development; their involvement will invariably facilitate implementation.

Drug acquisition costs change regularly. For example, patent expiry and generic drug manufacture at lower costs (as will happen to the 5-HT$_3$ receptor antagonists in the near future) can have profound cost implications. It is important that local costs are reviewed and changes made to PONV guidelines to reflect the most cost-effective use of resources as well as new evidence about clinical efficacy.

Education and monitoring

The drug prescription charts of nearly all patients in hospitals are scanned daily by pharmacists. This intensive monitoring makes a key contribution to risk management in hospital wards and gives an opportunity to evaluate and collect data on outcomes from changes in practice. For example, the effect of introducing new prescribing guidelines can be evaluated at the point of delivery of care with deviations from expected practice detected and rectified if necessary by informal guidance and advice at an early stage, often on a 'one-to-one' basis.

The nursing contribution

The traditional process for managing PONV is influenced strongly by a medical perspective. In this process, nursing staff are isolated from the assessment of risk and prevention of PONV. This part of the traditional PONV management process has largely been the domain of medical staff, usually anaesthetists. However, nursing staff now routinely work in surgical pre-assessment units and are responsible for delivering patient information and education. Unlike nursing professionals, medical staff usually have little involvement with the direct consequences of PONV (many will have observed the ability of a vomit bowl to isolate a nurse and retching patient). Nurses are usually responsible for the first line assessment of patients in wards, as well as for giving drugs and other non-pharmacological treatments. Further, clinical audit (and increasingly research) are becoming essential activities for many nursing posts. Hence, nursing staff have a pivotal role in the wider management of PONV. Ward nurses in particular are identified as key players. In summary:

- ward nurses represent a relatively stable population of the ward work force;
- are directly exposed, on a daily basis, to patients with pain and nausea;
- are typically involved in pre-admission unit patient assessments;

- have 24 hour responsibility for pre and post-operative patient management including pain and PONV monitoring;
- have a vested interest in improving pain and PONV management since these problems impact directly on their workload and the suffering they see.

Pre-operative assessment clinics

Pre-assessment clinics provide an ideal opportunity for nurses to improve PONV outcomes by initiating the management process. In our experience, nurses can routinely perform and document a PONV risk assessment and deliver patient information in the clinic (Figure 8.1). Nightingale (1994) suggested a structured questionnaire could be used to identify risk factors. We (like others) have used a simple, practical tool to stratify risk in specific patient groups whose PONV outcomes are well documented through repeated audit.

Patients may take opportunities at the pre-assessment clinic to express anxieties that they would otherwise avoid with other professional groups. Written information can be reinforced by simple 'testing' and giving the patient an opportunity for questions. In our experience, this use of nursing time is extremely valuable, ensuring that the information is understood and clarifying the roles and responsibilities of patients as well as staff. This can alter expectations, hopefully in a realistic manner. Jolley (2000a) suggests that *interactive* delivery of patient information about PONV should

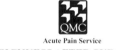

Acute Pain Service

SICKNESS AFTER SURGERY

Some people worry about feeling or being sick after an operation. This leaflet answers the questions that patients often ask.

Q. Is everyone sick after an operation?
A. No. Roughly one third of people feel sick, whilst two thirds usually don't.

Q. Are some people more likely to be sick than others?
A. Some people seem more sensitive to treatments than others. Also how long the operation takes, the sort of operation it is and which pain killers are used can have an effect.

Q. Can sickness be prevented?
A. Yes. There are drugs which can be given at the same time as the anaesthetic. It is important to tell the nurse or the anaesthetist of any worries you have. Before your operation they will ask you questions to see if you are more likely than usual to feel sick.

Q. Is it necessary to have an injection?
A. Not usually. We use a special needle for your anaesthetic which we leave in the back of your hand or arm to save jabbing you again.

Q. How long does the feeling of sickness last?
A. Everybody is different. Usually sickness soon passes off, especially once some treatment has been given.

Q. Can I do anything to avoid feeling sick?
A. Yes. After your operation try not to make sudden movements. When sitting up or getting out of bed, move slowly and smoothly.

When you start drinking take small sips and build up to proper drinking gradually. Eat small light meals to start with.

If you do feel sick, take slow deep breaths to reduce the sensation. Most importantly, tell a nurse as soon as you feel the slightest bit sick.

SIX TOP TIPS FOR COPING WITH SICKNESS

- Warn us if you've felt sick after other operations
- Tell a nurse straight away if you feel sick
- Move slowly and smoothly
- Drink small sips to begin with
- Eat little, light and often
- Try taking deep breaths if sickness strikes

REMEMBER

The staff at QMC understand how unpleasant it is to feel sick. We will do everything to prevent it. If you are unfortunate enough to suffer any sickness we will treat you promptly and give you privacy and support.

Developed for QMC patients
with the help of QMC patients

Source: Queen's Medical Centre, Nottingham

Figure 8.1 Patient PONV information leaflet.

become an integral part of general pre-operative advice. In our multi-cultural society, multi-lingual written and verbal patient information after consultation with relevant patient forums is desirable.

Prophylaxis, education and training

Without specific training, important gaps exist in nurses' knowledge about PONV (Jolley 2000b). This work suggests that identifying these gaps and delivering feedback to staff can help target training in an effective manner and increase staff motivation. Nurses with greater knowledge of the aetiology of PONV and anti-emetic drugs may make more informed decisions about treatments (Tate *et al.* 1996) and have a heightened awareness of the problem. Guidelines will almost certainly help this decision-making process.

Prompt treatment

Routine systematic assessment and recording of pain after surgery is mandatory; a similar attitude should be applied to the management of PONV. Without obsessive regular assessment, the patient may be reluctant to 'disturb' nursing staff and make their symptoms and requirements known. There are, however, several issues to consider before implementation. Some of these are outlined in Table 8.2. We consider that documentation of the nursing response to assessment is an essential part of improving outcomes by introducing some 'bedside accountability' with the documentation providing additional opportunity for subsequent clinical supervision and audit.

Table 8.2 Some considerations for PONV ward nursing policy

Does the ITU, recovery room and ward (and emergency department?) nurse monitoring chart include a section for recording PONV?

How often should PONV be assessed and recorded?

Who makes the assessments? (trained nurses, student nurses, healthcare assistants?)

Which rating method should be used?
    Nausea (Yes/no; none/mild/moderate/severe; numerical rating/visual analogue scale, duration?)
    Vomiting (Yes/no; number of episodes)
    Combination scales* (e.g. combining nausea and vomiting)

Should the nursing response to assessment be documented?

Time period after giving anti-emetic before re-assessment?

Definition of treatment failure? When and where to refer patient?

* Not recommended. Assessments of nausea and vomiting should be made independently.

The lack of access of a nurse (and therefore the patient) to an appropriate and evidence-based prescription is an important factor retarding improvement in PONV outcomes. The use of pre-printed anti-emetic prescription labels (Figure 8.2) on the drug prescription chart is one strategy improving access to drug treatments in the recovery room and wards. We allow the use of two different anti-emetics within 30 minutes of each other, as appropriate. This is consistent with the use of 'balanced anti-emesis' (Heffernan *et al.* 2000) for treating PONV and implies the need for timely, repeated assessment and treatment when necessary. There may, however, be implications for nursing practice and the use of nursing time.

QMC	Adult Anti-Emetic Treatment Prescription (2ⁿᵈ dose of Ondansetron can be given after 30 minutes)								
Acute Pain Service	Cyclizine 50 mg iv/im 8 hrly pro	Date Time Route Given				Ondansetron 4 mg iv/im	Date Time Route Given			Signed_____ Date / /

Source: Queen's Medical Centre, Nottingham

Figure 8.2 Pre-printed anti-emetic prescription label for treatment of PONV.

However, the use of aggressive drug treatment regimens must be reconciled with the wishes of the patient. Patients may have preferences for or against specific drug delivery modes. Nurses recognise that PONV may be dangerous in the immediate post-operative period, particularly in the recovery room, and that some patients express a preference to avoid PONV even if they must experience increased pain (Paech *et al.* 1998). On other occasions, witnessed PONV may be associated with feelings of embarrassment for the patients and some may wish to be given their privacy (Thompson 1999).

Non-pharmacological interventions

Although there is a lack of evidence, several nursing interventions may promote a holistic approach. Our local audit indicates that patients do consider some of these interventions desirable. For example, Thompson (1999) suggests the covers on the dietary tray should be removed away from the patient, allowing strong odours to dissipate before the tray is presented to the patient. Traditional teaching is that eating or drinking too soon after an operation might lead to PONV (Nightingale 1994). However a controlled, blinded trial comparing clear liquid diet to regular diet in 241 patients undergoing abdominal surgery found that PONV was not increased in patients who received a regular diet as their first post-operative meal (Jeffrey *et al.* 1996). This issue requires further investigation.

Patient privacy and dignity, nutrition and mouth care have been highlighted in the *Essence of Care* (Department of Health 2001) document as fundamental aspects of nursing care that require benchmarking. In relation to PONV management factors such as the use of screens, the provision of vomit bowls, tissues, mouth nasogastric aspiration trays should be considered.

Movement of patients, especially those with a history of motion sickness be smooth and slow (Nightingale 1994; Thompson 1999). Relaxation with guided imagery has not been shown to reduce the incidence of PONV but has been shown to be effective for reducing nausea in patients undergoing chemotherapy (Hawthorn 1995).

Many pain management specialist nurses have the skills to perform acupuncture and transcutaneous electrical nerve stimulation for pain relief. It is vital that non-pharmacological interventions for PONV are studied further if we are to avoid overlooking useful and simple therapeutic modalities; further research with other health professionals is required.

Short-stay surgical units and hospital-to-home

Doctors and nurses must increasingly balance a shortage of hospital beds with the timing of discharge after surgery. The timing of discharge may have a detrimental effect on patients' experiences of pain and nausea. A qualitative study explored patients' experiences of post-operative pain, nausea and vomiting (Waterman *et al.* 1999). Satisfaction and outcomes after discharge were extremely poor for many patients, although one patient stayed in a hotel with her family for two nights as this was preferable to staying in the hospital. The multidisciplinary team must consider the issue of outcomes after discharge when implementing any management strategy.

The role of clinical guidelines

Over recent years increasing numbers of clinical guidelines have been produced at both local and national levels. An approach to developing, appraising and applying clinical guidelines has been published by the NHS Executive (Mann 1996). Using these 'guidelines for guidelines' may be useful (Carter 1993). The Institute of Medicine defines clinical guidelines as 'systematically developed statements to assist practitioner and patient decisions about appropriate health care for specific clinical circumstances' (Field *et al.* 1990). The principal benefit should be to improve quality of patient care. An additional aim is to improve the consistency of care so that patients are treated in the same way regardless of where or by whom they are treated. For practitioners, guidelines clarify interventions of proven benefit and question ineffective or wasteful practices. However, guidelines should provide guidance rather than instructions or commands, and are therefore distinct from protocols.

Attempts to introduce clinical guidelines are often met with seasoned local scepticism. This response may be justified in many situations (Table 8.1; Rubin *et al.* 2000). There are legitimate concerns about the time and effort required to develop high quality guidelines, the variable quality of some existing guidelines, and the potential for suppressing innovation or patient-centred care by imposing a flawed guideline (Hopkins 1995). There is, however, potential for clinical guidelines to improve the quality of care. For example, implementation of guidelines may reduce length of hospital admission and drug costs resulting in value for money (Shapiro *et al.* 1993). However, local guideline implementation may fail to change clinical practice or to maintain changes if a sound process of development and implementation is neglected and inappropriately resourced, and the evidence base for effectiveness of implementation of strategies is ignored (Table 8.1). Too often excessive complexity, poor presentation, and poor organisation and management of the change process leads to ineffective guidelines.

Developing guidelines for managing PONV

In general, there may be three main components of usable guidelines (Jackson *et al.* 1998):

1. *Explicit identification of the key decisions relevant to patients and their consequences.* Flow diagrams or algorithms would seem to be appropriate (e.g. Figure 8.3).

2. *Review of the relevant, valid evidence on benefits, risks and costs of alternative decisions.* A succinct summary of evidence to aid decision-making in the PONV algorithm, including a shortlist of appropriate anti-emetics might be relevant and useful. Although good economic data relevant to PONV management is scarce, there are many reviews of current evidence in PONV management, in particular, the efficacies and adverse effects of anti-emetic drugs (Tramer 2001a). Tramer (2001b) has discussed the clinical actions required to achieve further PONV reduction. In addition to improving pharmacological prophylaxis and anti-emesis management, the reduction of baseline risk is highlighted.

3. *Accessible presentation to inform key decisions that is flexible to stakeholder preferences.* A simple, patient specific and user friendly format is desirable. The guideline should specify its aims and the target patient population. It should also clarify which health professionals should use the guidelines and who has been responsible for their development and ratification. A date for review of the guidelines is also desirable.

The key decisions in PONV management

There are two key areas for decision-making in PONV management. These are:

1. *Prevention.* What interventions are appropriate for the prevention of PONV in the individual patient?
2. *Treatment.* What interventions are appropriate for the treatment of PONV in the individual patient?

A. Prevention of PONV

There may be four components to the effective prophylaxis of PONV.

1. Patient preparation

Patient information is an integral part of any care pathway. Patients in our hospital have specifically regarded the provision of information as a useful strategy in PONV care. Our service finds a highly interactive nursing approach to delivering patient information particularly effective for changing patient expectations and knowledge. Verbal delivery reinforced with a written leaflet has been associated with successful outcomes. It is important to ask for feedback and 'test' patients, repeating the education as appropriate. Training of anaesthetists and other doctors may improve the use of intra-operative prophylaxis and post-operative prescribing, but without education of nursing staff and patients there is no guarantee that an appropriate anti-emetic prescription will be used effectively if at all.

2. Risk assessment

Assigning individual patient risk is the first decision in the PONV management pathway. This will allow the application of appropriate, specific interventions for prevention of PONV.

PONV has a well documented multifactorial aetiology, one of the reasons for previous failure to improve outcomes. During the pre-operative visit, it is common practice for anaesthetists to elicit risk factors such as previous PONV and motion sickness from the history, and to consider gender and post-operative opioid use. This assessment may be rooted in science, but most clinicians will then informally assign patients to receive either no prophylactic anti-emetic or prophylactic anti-emetic according to 'low' or 'high' risk. Some may now consider giving two prophylactic anti-emetics for 'higher' risk. There are no published data evaluating the effectiveness of this informal risk assessment and whether it is linked to appropriate and proportionate therapeutic responses for actual risk. It may therefore be better than nothing but no more than an educated, clinical 'hunch' with potential mismatch of therapeutic strategies and actual risk. Formal quantification of risk must be rare in everyday practice.

In order to improve the quality of risk assessment, the ability to assess risk simply and more accurately at the bedside is required. Initial models describing the relative importance of individual risk factors and their predictive value (e.g. Koivuranta *et al.* 1997) suggest complex formulae for estimating individual risk of developing PONV. Although useful in the research setting and confirming the relative importance of risk factors for clinicians, the application of these models to routine clinical practice is not practical. More recently this approach has been simplified (Apfel *et al.* 2002a; Gan 2002) so that the number of major risk factors (female gender, non-smoker status, history of PONV or motion sickness, post-operative opioid use) is totalled (Table 8.3). Risk of PONV increases dramatically, from 10% with none to approaching 80% with all four risk factors. This tool is simple and practical, allowing quantification of PONV risk at the bedside. Therapeutic strategies proportionate to the number of risk factors may then be developed and applied. There is no reason why this assessment cannot be performed by nursing staff, who may have a higher perception of risk of PONV than medical staff.

Table 8.3 Simplified risk score (after Apfel *et al.* 1998). (If none, one, two, three or four risk factors are present, the risk for PONV is approximately 10, 20, 40, 60 and 80% respectively.)

Risk factors	Points
Female gender	1
Non-smoking status	1
History of PONV and/or motion sickness	1
Post-operative opioids	1

Guidelines should improve assessment and clearly link risk to appropriate and proportionate interventions to be effective. However, the effect of guidelines on the process of risk assessment is not well documented. Our local audit suggests that the introduction of guidelines with a brief narrative simply encouraging a risk assessment, outlining risk factors, and recommending the use of a specified single prophylactic anti-emetic in patients with any risk factors can change practice. However, there remains little evidence of appropriate matching of proportionate therapy to risk; the effect on outcomes may be limited if subsequent patient PONV management during and after surgery is neglected.

3. Reduce the baseline risk

Tramer (2001b) highlights the reduction of baseline risk as an initial strategy before making decisions about other interventions. For example, a low baseline risk may not support a blanket approach to prophylaxis; a 'treatment only' strategy may be more cost-effective.

Should a 'prescription' for anaesthetic technique be part of PONV policy? The anaesthetic factors influencing PONV outcomes are well documented. In general, many of these factors have a relatively small influence on late PONV outcomes (after 2–6 hours). Tramer (2001b) concludes that three anaesthetic interventions have sufficient evidence for further consideration; use of propofol infusion (effect only on early PONV), omitting nitrous oxide and omitting larger doses of anti-cholinesterase to antagonise neuromuscular blockade. More recently, the use of volatile agents has been identified as a major factor producing early PONV (the first 2 hours) (Apfel *et al.* 2002b).

Choosing these less emetogenic anaesthetic interventions together with better (non-opioid) pain management techniques and less invasive surgical techniques may reduce baseline frequency of PONV. All anaesthetists should be aware of these factors and local training initiatives are therefore important. Thereafter, local outcomes and consensus should determine how prescriptive PONV policy is toward individual anaesthetic technique.

4. Pharmacological intervention

The evidence base for prophylaxis of PONV suggests pharmacological intervention is appropriate. However, the gap between outcomes from a carefully controlled research study and translating this into everyday practice are easily appreciated by clinical staff. Information from systematic reviews and from other chapters in this book will be invaluable when choosing specific drug interventions for prevention of PONV. There are, however a number of issues to consider after implementing measures to reduce baseline risk and assessing individual patient risk.

- *Is there a role for routine drug prophylaxis?* Debate about the use of routine anti-emetic prophylaxis has been ongoing for over 40 years (Adriani *et al.* 1961). Opinion will differ according to the perspective. The patient's perspective might overwhelmingly be in favour of routine prophylaxis (particularly those with a past history of PONV), as PONV has been regarded by patients as equally distressing as pain (Tsui *et al.* 1997). However, many patients will receive unnecessary prophylaxis and there will be more adverse events and greater direct costs. This may be offset by a smaller demand on ward nursing time. On the other hand, consideration of only direct drug costs may discourage the use of prophylaxis, especially with the more expensive anti-emetic drugs. A wider consideration of cost-effectiveness suggests a more limited role for prophylaxis according to the baseline risk of PONV; for ondansetron, treatment is more cost-effective than routine prophylaxis (Tramer 1999). Risk quantification, the expected baseline frequency of PONV, the potential for other adverse sequelae from vomiting, and what 'works' in the local clinical environment will ultimately influence local policy. Further work to evaluate the cost-effectiveness of combination prophylaxis is required.

- *What drugs should be recommended for prophylaxis?* Which anti-emetics should be used in different clinical situations? Is one drug better for preventing nausea and another for vomiting? Should a single or combination approach be adopted? When should anti-emetics be given during surgery?
    The literature now provides considerable evidence to help answer these questions. Some of these data are outlined in other chapters of this book. Single agent prophylaxis has little to recommend it as it is not particularly effective

compared with combination prophylaxis. Combination anti-emetic prophylaxis with drugs having different mechanisms of action can markedly reduce the incidence of PONV. Under research conditions, ondansetron and cyclizine can achieve a response rate of 95% (Ahmed *et al.* 2000). Similar efficacy has been reported for a 5-HT$_3$ receptor antagonist and either droperidol (McKenzie *et al.* 1996) or dexamethasone (Fujii *et al.* 1995). It is unfortunate that droperidol has now been withdrawn from the UK (risk of cardiac arrthymias or QT$_c$ interval prolongation) as it is probably the most evidence-based prophylactic anti-emetic and relatively good for preventing nausea.

Multimodal therapy taken to the extreme incorporating propofol and combination anti-emetics has produced a 98% complete response rate (Scuderi *et al.* 2000), although cost-effectiveness requires further consideration. As there is no such thing as pre-emptive anti-emesis, prophylaxis should be given shortly before extubation/emergence (Henzi *et al.* 2000).

B. Treatment of PONV

There are perhaps three elements to consider when developing clinical guidelines for treating PONV; pharmacological intervention, treatment failure and organisational issues.

1. Pharmacological intervention

The issues are similar to those for pharmacological prophylaxis.

• *Is there a role for routine anti-emetic prescription?* There is no doubt that all patients should have an anti-emetic prescribed for use after surgery. However, prescribing may be erratic and traditional. A clinical guideline must consider methods to influence and optimise prescribing. There is an important role for education but additional strategies can be useful. Our experience using 'reminders' such as pre-printed 'sticky' labels (Figure 8.2) suggests that this can be a successful strategy. This simplifies the prescribing process for anaesthetic and ward staff and improves nursing and therefore patient access to treatment with anti-emetics. This method does not seek to remove clinical choice when prescribing anti-emetics, as the clinician may choose another prescription. However, it can significantly change drug use as it has done in our institution. For example, the use of metoclopramide, an anti-emetic with a relatively poor evidence-base for the treatment of PONV, has been marginalised using this technique.

• *Which anti-emetics should be used? Are complementary therapies efficacious?* Although much work has been published on PONV prophylaxis, the number of trials reporting treatment outcomes for established PONV is limited. This is most likely the result of the large numbers of patients required and the logistical difficulties with trial design. The most efficacious intervention in PONV treatment is ondansetron (Tramer *et al.* 1997b). For all other interventions there is a relative lack of data.

• *Single or combination therapy? What is a reasonable time between treatments should the first fail?* Unlike prophylaxis, there is a lack of data for combination therapy in the treatment of established PONV. Again, the logistical difficulties with trial design are one cause. Some unpublished data from our study of 200 patients with established nausea and/or vomiting in the recovery room after a variety of operations may be relevant. Patients were randomised to receive either ondansetron or cyclizine in a double blind manner, followed by crossover treatment at 30 minutes if the first treatment had failed. These data indicated that ondansetron was the most efficacious anti-emetic, with significantly less patients requiring rescue (crossover) treatment at 30 minutes (24% vs 39%). However, there was only one patient in the study who had persistent PONV requiring further treatment at 60 minutes after the first treatment. These data may support the use of combination treatment; it would be interesting to establish the need for rescue treatment at 30 minutes had both drugs been given simultaneously.

There is insufficient pharmacokinetic/dynamic data to make sound recommendations for the minimum interval between treatments. Our 2002 national survey suggests one hour is a common recommendation in practice; we recommend 30 minutes after intravenous treatment. In the absence of good evidence, it seems reasonable to prescribe more than one anti-emetic for treatment and to give these simultaneously or at least in quick succession as appropriate. This has implications for nursing policy and the nursing perspective must be considered. For example, the choice of an anti-emetic with an intravenous formulation may enhance nursing practice, patients' perception of care (and probably the onset of action) compared to intramuscular injections.

2. Treatment failure

It should be clear to nursing staff that it is not sufficient to give an anti-emetic and accept a poor outcome. Criteria for 'treatment failure' and the expected course of action must be explicit and subject to audit. This is an issue for local consensus.

3. Organisational issues

The implementation of an active, responsive, patient-centred policy for treatment of PONV has clear implications for the organisation of recovery and ward nursing care. There are obvious training, documentation and support issues.

Are guidelines for PONV management used in the UK?

In 2002, we surveyed 200 UK institutions in order to assess the use of guidelines and provision of patient information, post-operative assessment and treatment for PONV management. Clinical directors or lead clinicians/nurses of acute pain services were asked to return a questionnaire about local PONV management together with a copy of any relevant clinical guidelines or algorithms. We received 102 replies (51% response rate). Table 8.4 gives some of the survey results.

Table 8.4 Data from a survey of PONV management in UK hospitals in 2002. Data are percentages of all replies (102 replies from 200 hospitals; all regions, district general and teaching hospitals represented).

Named person with responsibility for PONV management	44
Have a formal 'guideline/policy'	46
Formal training of nursing staff	64
Provide patient information*	62
Verbal only	43
Written leaflet only	9
Use prescribing guidelines	52
Use metoclopramide for either prophylaxis and/or prevention	36
Post-operative assessment of PONV	87
Both nausea & vomiting	76
Document assessment	84
Use non-pharmacological/complementary treatments	31

* About one-third of patients receiving information do so from the anaesthetist.

Clearly there was substantial interest in the use of guidelines for PONV management. The majority focused on the treatment of PONV, the area of PONV management with the least evidence base. It was apparent that cost was driving the choice of drugs for treatment and not evidence as 5-HT$_3$ antagonists were assigned to a second or often third rank after other anti-emetics, including metoclopramide. A common aim was to assess and treat PONV within a one hour period, with referral of treatment failures after two or three 'cycles' of treatment.

Guidelines for prophylaxis were often absent or non-specific, despite there being much more data available about this aspect of PONV management. Similarly, the use of formal risk assessment was infrequent.

The use of clinical audit

Why audit PONV?

Audit of clinical guidelines is a potential weakness for a variety of reasons, not least for lack of appropriate resources. Some may find it irksome. It may also be assumed that local guidelines are improving clinical effectiveness and therefore substitute for clinical audit. This may discourage the application of audit and jeopardise effective development, implementation and monitoring of policy. However, guidelines and recommended pathways of care can provide the ideal structure for effective audit (West *et al.* 1997). Information via clinical audit with appropriate feedback is fundamental to any policy attempting to change clinical practice and outcomes and verify application of guidelines and policy. It is important to the development and implementation process as well as more obviously the monitoring and maintenance of clinical practice and outcomes.

Audit during policy development

Unless the baseline risk is known, it is impossible to know whether any intervention has had the desired effect. It may be difficult to assign appropriate prophylaxis. Documentation of PONV outcomes may be useful for raising awareness and justifying the use of staff time in development.

Audit during policy implementation

Few anaesthetists, ward staff or patients will have an accurate knowledge of the incidence of PONV in their area of work. There is usually little local examination of the process and outcomes from PONV management other than isolated and infrequent audit projects. Are patients adequately assessed for risk of PONV and is prophylaxis used appropriately? Have all post-operative patients an evidence-based anti-emetic prescription available and how is it used? Without a continuous audit programme and appropriate dissemination of results there will be neither appreciation of the need for change nor ammunition to bring about such change.

Audit for monitoring of policy

Maintaining policy and guideline effectiveness is challenging. Audit is fundamental to this challenge. It can detect changing practice. For example, we have detected a substantial drift in the use of treatment recommendations from the first line to the second line anti-emetic recommendation. Coincidentally, evidence is now available to support this practice change.

Improving audit effectiveness

The audit process is well documented; the specific characteristics of an effective audit process are less so. The frequency of audit, the relevance of the dataset and the feedback process should at least be considered. For example, the incidence of PONV is well documented in the literature and resources are scarce. Therefore intermittent audit targeting areas of clinical concern may be most practical. However, local outcomes may vary considerably in response to the changing local organisation. Continuous audit will confirm that guidelines are being used, provide routine feedback about patient outcomes and detect aberrations allowing for their rectification in a timely manner. This may be more likely to promote and maintain outcome improvements.

In practice, few institutions will be able to resource a continuous audit mechanism for PONV management. Regular, intermittent sampling using snapshot or cohort techniques may be useful. An alternative includes embedding the audit process in the day to day management of PONV by delegating responsibility to ward nurses, requiring nurses to audit other wards and feed back data at regular intervals. This may have a secondary effect of ensuring that nursing documentation of ward PONV management is of a higher standard. It should also be possible to give patients a continuous invitation for feedback on outcomes, perhaps as part of the ward discharge process.

Pharmacy departments may make additional contributions to audit. In addition to ward-based surveillance, pharmacy information systems can produce detailed, hospital-wide information on the use and costs of various types of drugs such as anti-emetics These data can be used to evaluate not only the effect of prescribing recommendations but also give a pre-audit indication of probable clinical outcomes. The pharmacy network can therefore provide a more continuous and realistic picture of practice outcomes than the impressions of clinical staff who have an intermittent presence on wards and who are primarily focused on each individual patient's care.

An effective audit process and clinical policy will be aided by the existence of dedicated funding. This must be a rare occurrence. Direct drug costs will usually be assimilated into a surgical or anaesthetic drug budget. There are no externally recognised 'targets' or 'waiting lists' for PONV management (although all surgical patients potentially constitute such a 'waiting list'). In practice, this means there is little chance of attracting additional dedicated resources for improving PONV care without building these into surgical funding bids, a similar situation to that of post-operative pain management. The required resources, largely staff time, usually come from within acute pain teams or anaesthetic departments. However, audit may have an important role in future retention or attraction of resources.

What are appropriate outcome measures?

A crucial decision determining the effectiveness and impact of audit is the choice of outcome measures or performance indicators. Two broad groups of measures, process and outcomes, are probably required to document the quality of PONV management. This dataset may also allow comparison between different institutions, although additional data such as casemix will be necessary.

Auditing the process

Table 8.5 gives a set of questions providing a simple yes/no assessment of the process for managing PONV. This is a descriptive dataset giving little indication of effectiveness. It should however be useful for benchmarking local policies for PONV management. Each of the factors can be audited in greater detail. For example, audit of staff knowledge of both PONV management and of the actual existence and use of relevant guidelines, and details of the ward organisation of PONV treatment will provide further insight. However, only patient outcome data will provide true evidence of policy application and effectiveness.

Table 8.5 Auditing the PONV management process

---

1. Is there an institutional/local policy for managing PONV?

2. Is there evidence of the following?

    A patient information/education instrument
    An instrument for assessing patient risk of PONV
    A strategy for targeting prophylaxis
    A strategy for treatment
    A strategy for managing persistent PONV

3. Is there a continuous education programme for staff managing PONV?

4. Is there specific policy for nursing observation, documentation and intervention for PONV?

5. Is there a clinical audit process?

Auditing patient outcomes

We highlight a number of relevant outcome measures after appraisal of published recommendations (e.g. Apfel *et al.* 2002a; Tramer 2001b), expert opinion, a survey of key clinical staff in UK institutions and our own experience with auditing these outcomes. We have considered practical issues and both staff and patient perspectives. Our interpretation of this consensus is given in Table 8.6. Clinical outcome measures are summarised as either essential or additional.

Nausea and vomiting have different pathophysiological mechanisms and should therefore be quantified individually (Tramer 2001b). The incidence of both, and the severity of nausea, are generally agreed to be essential PONV outcomes. Short-term outcomes (from 2 to 6 hours after surgery) may have an economic impact in day surgery or recovery rooms; presence of PONV may necessitate overnight hospital admission with a dramatic increase in the cost of the procedure, or delay discharge from recovery. Longer-term efficacy, up to 24 or more hours after operation, may influence a patient's outcomes on the journey home or at home.

Table 8.6 Clinical (patient) outcome measures for PONV management. (Patients rate severity/duration of nausea as less acceptable than vomiting.)

Essential (early and late for each of the following e.g. 0–2h, 2–24h)	
Nausea	Incidence (%)
	Severity[1]
	Duration[2]
Vomiting	Incidence (%)
	Number of episodes
Nausea and/or vomiting or	
Complete response[3]	Incidence (%)
Escape/rescue treatment[4]	Incidence (%)
Patient satisfaction[5]	

Additional
Delay until first episode of nausea and/or vomiting
Timing of each episode of vomiting (for survival analysis)
Time to readiness for discharge (from recovery or day surgery unit) or did PONV
  delay discharge? (from recovery or day surgery unit; nurse assessment; yes/no)
Adverse events: yes or no[6]

[1] Mild, moderate or severe; numerical rating scale (NRS, 0–10).
[2] E.g. ordinal scale (Likert; <1h, 1–2h, 2–4h, >4h), derive from nursing chart.
[3] No nausea or vomiting.
[4] Patients requiring at least one treatment.
[5] Global rating for 24 h or for specific aspects of care e.g. patient information, treatment response, need to improve care of PONV (yes/no).
[6] E.g. headache, restlessness, sedation, dry mouth.

What audit of PONV is performed in UK practice?

In our 2002 survey (Table 8.4), 68% of the 102 hospitals that replied stated that PONV audit was performed in their hospital; the APS performed the audit in 71% of these hospitals and 20% performed daily audit. An additional 70% performed intermittent audit at least every 12 months. Forty five percent considered continuous monitoring desirable.

What can be achieved by implementing a policy for PONV management?

Published data

There is limited published evidence evaluating the role of policy changes, clinical guidelines and audit for improving PONV outcomes. Hadji *et al.* (1998) suggested that PONV incidence could be reduced from 71.5% to approaching 51% following the introduction of a departmental policy for PONV management. Other papers suggest that guidelines can change practice, improve care and reduce costs (Busch

1996, Nolte *et al.*1998). Another study involving over 2700 patients in 15 hospitals throughout the UK introduced education for both staff and patients with formal pain assessment and a standardised prescription for post-operative pain management. This was associated with a reduced incidence of moderate and severe nausea or vomiting by 14% and 10% respectively (Harmer *et al.* 1998). Following unacceptably high rates of pain and nausea, changes in institutional practice reduced pain scores, but nausea scores remained unchanged (Stockdale *et al.* 1998).

Unpublished data (local audit)

We, like many others, have put together 'guidelines' for PONV management. Our serial attempts to improve outcomes in patients after gynaecological surgery have provided useful local data and lessons for policy development and implementation.

Guidelines, audit and a 'sticky label'

In 1996, we distributed a simple set of guidelines for PONV management to anaesthetists and nursing staff in the recovery room, and also displayed laminated versions in anaesthetic rooms and the recovery area. The guidelines were similar to many of those received in our 2002 UK survey. The guidelines were directed toward anaesthetists and encouraged an informal risk assessment, recommending the use of prophylactic intravenous cyclizine in patients with risk factors for PONV. The guidelines focused attention on better prescribing of anti-emetics for the treatment of established PONV through the use of pre-printed anti-emetic prescription labels (Figure 8.2). Nursing colleagues in recovery and the wards were encouraged to monitor PONV more closely, with the anti-emetic prescription protocol giving them the opportunity to administer doses of two different anti-emetics within 30 minutes of each other if appropriate.

Extensive audit demonstrated the patient cohorts before and after guideline implementation to have comparable demographic, risk, intraoperative and pain data. There was a significant increase (from approximately 20% to 40%) in the number of patients receiving prophylaxis and a significant change in the prophylactic anti-emetic given to cyclizine. Use of the prescription labels by anaesthetists increased the availability of two anti-emetics for treating PONV from 3% to 80% of patients. There were clinical improvements associated with these clear changes in anti-emetic prescription and administration. These included a modest reduction in PONV in recovery and a reduction in the number of patients recording moderate or severe nausea in the first 24 hours after surgery. A similar reduction in the number of patients receiving anti-emetics on wards (despite more reliable nursing access to appropriate anti-emetic prescriptions) suggested that this change was the result of better prophylaxis and treatment in operating theatres. However, subsequent audits in 1998 all demonstrated an ongoing problem with PONV. The overall incidence of vomiting during the first post-operative 24 hours persisted at around 25%. Further, there was some 'drift' in the choice of anti-emetic for prophylaxis to ondansetron with cost implications for the anaesthetic drug budget.

A comprehensive, multidisciplinary policy. Worth the additional effort?

Our APS decided to address these problems by incorporating the existing guidelines and PONV treatment protocol into a comprehensive PONV management strategy. A proposal was submitted to and approved by the local Ethics Committee. The key aims of the project included the following.

- To develop a comprehensive management policy to improve PONV outcomes for patients and staff,
- To evaluate this policy.

a. Methods

Specific clinical areas were identified for participation in the project; the pre-assessment clinics, operating department, recovery room and two gynaecology wards. Two staff nurses from the gynaecology wards were seconded part-time to the project for one year. They were fully involved in all data collection and analysis, developing the required documentation and participating in the education programme. Most importantly, because they were still working on their wards they were able to act as opinion leaders and influence the rate of uptake of change by ward nursing and medical colleagues (Bury 1998).

The project was divided into three phases:

Phase 1. Preliminary clinical audit to establish current standards of management and to determine patients' expectations, beliefs and preferences in relation to PONV. Data were collected before surgery, at the time of discharge from the recovery room, at 24 and 48 hours after surgery, and at the time of hospital discharge. These data were used to develop the documentation required in the second phase of the project as well as document clinical standards. There was an emphasis on the patients' perspective throughout the questionnaires.

Phase 2. Development of the management policy and supporting documentation. This included:

- a patient information leaflet developed with patients and piloted before implementation (Figure 8.1);
- information/educational tools for theatre and ward nursing/medical staff;
- a simple nurse-led PONV risk assessment tool (yes/no answers to four questions about well known risk factors; yes to any one classified the patient as high risk as all patients were female);
- anti-emetic prescribing guidelines for both prophylaxis and treatment (Figures 8.4 and 8.2 respectively);
- a patient satisfaction questionnaire for regular use in everyday clinical practice;

- education of all staff involved in implementing the change;
- implementation of the policy and supporting processes after consultation with relevant staff.

Figure 8.3 gives an algorithm summarising the clinical pathway. This was used as a basis for educating staff and patients and making responsibilities clear. Table 8.7 outlines these responsibilities.

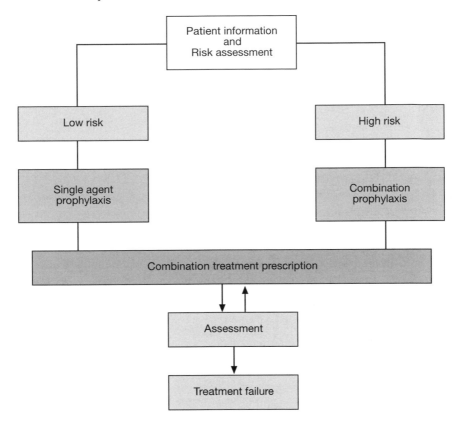

Figure 8.3 Algorithm for PONV management.

Adult Prophylactic Anti-Emetic Prescription. For anaesthetist use only. Give prophylaxis according to risk.
See QMC Acute Pain Service Adult PONV protocol for gynaecology

		Time	Given			Time	Given	Signed _____
Low risk ☐	Cyclizine 50mg iv			High risk ☐	Cyclizine 50mg iv &			
					Ondansetron 4mg iv			Date / /

Source: Queen's Medical Centre, Nottingham

Figure 8.4 Pre-printed label for risk assessment and recommended prophylactic anti-emetics.

Table 8.7 PONV policy: staff and patient responsibilities

Patients: Read the written patient information and ask questions where appropriate. Be aware of the treatments available, who can give these and when these may be given. Expect to be assessed at regular intervals and to notify nursing staff if there are problems with feeling or being sick. Expect to receive prompt treatment, when requested.

Gynaecology ward nurses: Undertake pre-operative risk assessment; identify high risk patients, educate patients pre-operatively and support this with the information leaflet; continue to monitor PONV and implement the treatment prescription; refer treatment failure.

Anaesthetists: reinforce information given by ward nurses; give prophylactic anti-emetic therapy according to identified risk; endorse the treatment prescription (sticky label); act as an information resource and medical support for ward colleagues.

Operating department practitioners: support and reinforce the implementation of the policy with anaesthetist colleagues.

Recovery room nurses: reinforce information given by ward nurses; continue to monitor PONV and implement the treatment prescription.

Ward based medical staff: support the policy, treat/refer treatment failure.

Physiotherapists: inform ward nurses if patients are unable to comply with therapy because of PONV.

APS specialist nurses: education and support of all staff, respond as soon as possible to treatment failure, implement alternative strategies, seek anaesthetic advice as appropriate.

Ward pharmacist: daily review of anti-emetic prescription; inform ward nurses if patient considers PONV therapy not effective.

Phase 3. Subsequent clinical audit to evaluate the effects of the management changes. This audit repeated the data collection of Phase 1.

b. Results

The two patient cohorts had comparable demographic, PONV risk, intra-operative and pain data. Table 8.8 gives some of the data from the audits performed before and after policy implementation. There were significant improvements in outcomes by incorporating guidelines into a multifaceted, multidisciplinary policy. In particular, there was a significant reduction in the severity and duration of nausea. The data demonstrate what may be achieved with a multidisciplinary policy, and what might be realistic targets or standards for PONV management in this patient group. Although there were some significant and clinically important improvements, outcomes approached rather than replicated those in published randomised trials.

Table 8.8 Results from PONV policy implementation. Data are percentages.

		Before *n = 140*	*After* *n = 150*
Formal risk assessment		–	100
Patient information (patient recall)		–	86
Received prophylactic anti-emetic		41	93
Recovery room			
Nausea	All	34	9
	Moderate or severe	18	5
Vomiting		7	2
Delayed discharge due to PONV		13	2
First 24 hours			
Nausea	All	58	28
	Moderate or severe	41	15
Vomiting		26	11

Patient assessment of policy outcomes. What are acceptable risks and experiences? In addition, there were significant changes in patient expectations and satisfaction. Five point Likert scales, simple yes/no statements and numerical rating scales (0–10) were used. For example, when asked if they expected to feel sick after their operation, 47% and 45% stated 'yes' both before and after policy implementation. However, 36% and 73% of patients before and after policy implementation respectively stated that they experienced much less sickness than expected. Further, 88% and 26% of patients before and after policy implementation respectively agreed with the statement that it was important that we improve the care of PONV.

At the time of hospital discharge, patients were asked a number of questions to help define 'acceptable' outcomes. There were some obvious differences associated with their PONV experience and significant changes in these preferences after policy implementation. However, the data for the second group (after policy implementation) as a whole gives some indication of the patient perspective and possible targets or standards for future PONV policy.

When asked to consider an acceptable risk for actual vomiting in the first 24 hours after surgery, 20% of patients stated that the risk should be ≤20%. However, 70% of patients stated that a risk ≥50% was acceptable. When asked to consider an acceptable risk for mild nausea (from a four point scale none, mild, moderate or severe), all patients stated this to be ≥50%. However, when asked to consider moderate or severe nausea only 11% of patients stated that they could tolerate this intensity of nausea for any time. Clearly, patients as a group regard more severe levels of nausea as undesirable and that vomiting and mild nausea are better tolerated. Most risk assessments focus on the frequency of vomiting, although patients are telling us that the reduction of moderate and severe nausea is their priority.

Given that it is unrealistic to abolish nausea, patients were then asked to consider if they were to experience nausea, what was an 'acceptable' duration quantified in hours; 65% stated this to be less than one hour, 28% 1–2 hours and 6% 2–4 hours. When asked to consider if they were to experience moderate or severe nausea, 91% and 7% stated that an 'acceptable' duration was less than one hour and 1–2 hours respectively.

Although crude, these data provide some targets for PONV policy from the patient perspective. We noted that in general, patients had a reduction in their tolerance for PONV after policy implementation. This may have been the result of higher expectations driven by the patient information tools and an improved PONV experience. Understandably, many patients preferred zero tolerance. This has implications for the delivery of patient information and adjustment of expectations to a more realistic outcome.

What is best practice?

Table 8.9 summarises the key components of best practice. Audit of local policy using suggested outcome measures (Tables 8.5 and 8.6) will give an indication of the quality of local PONV management. Our 2002 UK survey results suggested a consensus that all institutions should have a comprehensive policy for PONV management (Table 8.5). However, there was considerable variation in opinion about what standards should be set for patient outcomes from PONV management. The Royal College of Anaesthetists publication (2000) 'Raising the Standard' provides audit recipes for PONV and gives some suggestions for these standards. However, our opinion is these standards for patient outcomes are a matter for local consideration until such time as national recommendations are put forward.

Table 8.9 Best practice. Key components of a PONV policy.

Multidisciplinary patient care	
Prevention of PONV	Patient preparation/information
	Risk assessment
	Reduce the baseline risk
	Pharmacological intervention
Treatment of PONV	Pharmacological intervention (routine, evidence based anti-emetic prescription)
	Strategy for treatment failure
	Effective organisation of ward PONV management
Staff training policy	
Audit policy	

After reviewing our local audit results including patient preferences, current published evidence and expert opinion, and the opinion of clinical staff from UK hospitals, we suggest a modification of our previous algorithm for PONV management (Figure 8.3). The modified algorithm excludes a role for single anti-emetic prophylaxis and treatment as a first line response (Figure 8.5).

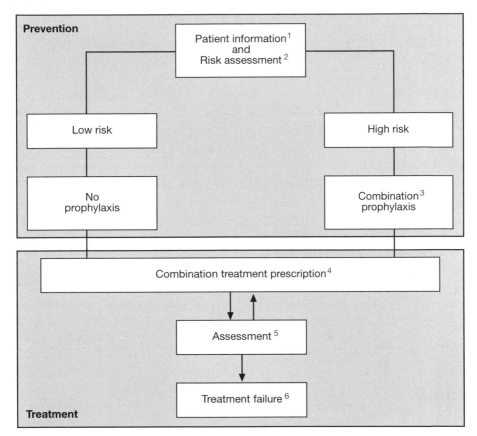

1. Patients should be informed about the care pathway, their risk assessment, and their responsibilities. An interactive approach supported by written information and confirmation of patient understanding is desirable.
2. See Table 8.3. The criteria for 'high risk' are variable and may be defined locally. A risk of at least 20% may be an appropriate starting point in the absence of good cost-effectiveness data. Patients rate moderate and severe nausea of any duration as their priority for management.
3. Combinations of a 5-HT$_3$ antagonist (preferably long acting) with either cyclizine, dexamethasone (or haloperidol?) may be appropriate.
4. Appropriate combinations for treatment will depend on prior prophylaxis and the time elapsed since prophylaxis.
    a) No prior prophylaxis: give a 5-HT$_3$ antagonist together with either cyclizine or prochlorperazine (IV route unavailable);
    b) Prior prophylaxis: give two anti-emetics with complementary modes of action. Consider repeating drugs used for prophylaxis (particularly a 5-HT$_3$ antagonist if an appropriate time interval has passed).
5. Nursing assessment, documentation and treatment should be efficient. Patients rate speed of response highly.
6. 'Treatment failure' and subsequent action require local definition. Most patients consider moderate or severe nausea for greater than 1–2 hours as unacceptable.

Figure 8.5 Updated algorithm for PONV management.

Some important issues to consider when implementing the algorithm

A key consideration in the algorithm is what is 'high' risk. This will depend on the perspective. Tramer (1997a) has suggested that the worthwhile efficacy of anti-emetic prophylaxis is arbitrarily defined as a number-needed-to-treat less than five. The baseline risk would need to be at least 20% to achieve this and thus 20% or greater might be regarded as high risk. This is based on the risk of vomiting.

However, in our experience, a majority of patients rate prevention of nausea as a higher priority than prevention of vomiting. Our audit indicates that patients wish to avoid moderate and severe nausea (using a four point ordinal scale) and will generally tolerate mild nausea. Perhaps then, PONV policy should consider risk of moderate or severe nausea and its duration as the primary outcome measure. (This suggests that anti-emetics with greatest efficacy for nausea such as droperidol or possibly haloperidol should be a part of a prophylactic or treatment anti-emetic policy.)

Some data from economic evaluations of PONV management are available in the literature. Although these data are useful, much of this work is based on the use of single drug prophylaxis and treatment. There is a clear need to conduct economic evaluations from different perspectives, using combination pharmacological strategies, to verify appropriate interventions for different baseline risks. At the present time, the criteria for defining low and high risk is probably best left to local judgement.

Most patients indicate that moderate and severe nausea should be resolved within one hour, and certainly two hours. This is a tight time schedule in busy wards and supports that use of combination anti-emetic treatment, with a rapid assessment and treatment cycle and identification of treatment failure by no later than two hours.

What attributes do patients consider important when rating the quality of PONV management in hospitals?

We asked 50 patients (who had experienced PONV) to consider themselves part of a hypothetical patient team with a remit to visit hospitals and rate the quality of PONV management, in particular, state the factors that would influence their judgement. Overwhelmingly, the most important factor was the actual presence and immediate availability of nurses in wards to help patients. Other factors included if nurses regularly asked if patients felt sick, had time to listen and actually offered treatment; the speed of response to requests for treatment; the provision of bowls, tissues and privacy; information before surgery about availability of treatment; and a strategy for prevention of PONV. Clearly the majority of concerns are about the organisation and effectiveness of nursing treatment on wards and not the actual frequency of PONV! (These issues have been discussed earlier in this chapter.) However, one study has shown that patients are prepared to pay much more than 10 times the cost of the most expensive anti-emetics for a complete response (Gan *et al.* 2001).

Conclusion

Although PONV research evidence is largely concerned with pharmacological options, the use of combination anti-emetic prophylaxis and treatment is an obvious and key component of PONV management policy. A pragmatic policy must also consider the overall system of delivering PONV care. The management of PONV may be considered analogous to post-operative pain management; poor organisation is the foundation for poor outcomes. The organisation and perspective of peri-operative care often gives PONV management a low priority with a lack of appreciation of the patient's perspective. The success of a new clinical policy will depend on effective contributions from all staff making relevant clinical decisions and delivering patient care throughout the surgical or PONV 'pathway'. The contributions of anaesthetists, pharmacists and nursing staff are therefore crucial. Resourcing the policy also requires consideration.

A key factor underpinning the success of clinical policy implementation, maintaining the policy and its associated clinical improvements, as well as obtaining and securing appropriate resources is the ability to demonstrate changes and associated outcomes. A comprehensive policy to re-organise PONV management must be multifaceted and include a multi-disciplinary approach, the use of clinical guidelines to get research evidence into practice, defining key decisions and improving the outcomes from these decisions, and the use of clinical audit. Future research should take a more pragmatic direction and evaluate daily practice and whole clinical regimens or packages with an emphasis on cost-effectiveness and the patient perspective.

References

Adriani, J., Summers, F.W., Antony, S.O. (1961). Is the prophylactic use of antiemetics in surgical patients justified? *Journal of the American Medical Association* **175**, 666–671.

Ahmed, A.B., Hobbs, G.J., Curran, J.P. (2000). Randomized, placebo-controlled trial of combination antiemetic prophylaxis for day-case gynaecological laparoscopic surgery. *British Journal of Anaesthesia* **85**, 678–682.

Apfel, C.C., Greim, C.A., Haubitz, I., Usadel, J., Sefrin, P., Roewer, N. (1998). A risk score to predict the probability of postoperative vomiting in adults. *Acta Anaesthesiologica Scandanavica* **42**, 495–501.

Apfel, C.C., Roewer, N., Korttila, K. (2002a). How to study postoperative nausea and vomiting. *Acta Anaesthesiologica Scandanavica* **46**, 921–928.

Apfel, C.C., Kranke, P., Katz, M.H., Goepfert, C., Papenfuss, T., Rauch, S., Heineck, R., Greim, C.A., Roewer, N. (2002b). Volatile anaesthetics may be the main cause of early but not delayed postoperative vomiting: a randomised controlled trial of factorial design. *British Journal of Anaesthesia* **88**, 659–668.

Association of Anaesthetists of Great Britain and Ireland (1998) *The Anaesthesia Team.*

Audit Commission (1997). Anaesthesia under examination. Audit Commission Publications, Abingdon, UK.

Bero, L.A., Grilli, R., Grimshaw, J.M., Harvey, E., Oxman, A.D., Thomson, M.A. (1998). Closing the gap between research and practice: an overview of systematic reviews of interventions to promote the implementation of research findings. *British Medical Journal* **317**, 465–468.

Bury, T. (1998). Getting research into practice. *in Evidence-based Healthcare: A Practical Guide for Therapists* (eds T Bury and J Mead), Butterworth Heinemann, Oxford.

Busch, A.F., Pearce, M.J., Allen, B. *et al.* (1996). Compliance with guidelines results in appropriate ondansetron prescribing at Christchurch Hospital. *New Zealand Medical Journal* **109**, 142–144.

Campbell, H., Hotchkiss, R., Bradshaw, N. *et al.* (1998). Integrated care pathways. *British Medical Journal* **316**, 133–137.

Carter, A. (1993). Background to the "guidelines for guidelines" series. *Canadian Medical Association Journal* **148**, 383.

Cohen, M.M., Duncan, P.G., De Boer, D.P., Tweed, W.A. (1994). The postoperative interview: assessing risk factors for nausea and vomiting. *Anesthesia and Analgesia* **78**, 7–16.

Davis, D.A., Thomson, M.A., Oxman, A.D., Haynes, R.B. (1995). Changing physician performance: a systematic review of the effect of educational strategies. *Journal of the American Medical Association* **274**, 700–705.

Department of Health (2001). The Essence of Care: Patient-Focused Benchmarking for Health Care Practitioners. Department of Health.

Field, M.J., Lohr, K.N. (eds) (1990). *Clinical practice guidelines: directions for a new program.* Washington, DC: National Academy Press.

Fisher, D.M. (1997). The 'big little problem' of postoperative nausea and vomiting (Editorial). *Anaesthesiology* **87**, 1271–1272.

Fulton, Y. (1997). Nurses' views on empowerment: a critical social theory perspective. *Journal of Advanced Nursing* **26**, 529–536.

Fujii, Y., Tanaka, H., Toyooka, H. (1995). Granisetron-dexamethasone combination reduces postoperative nausea and vomiting. *Canadian Journal of Anaesthesia* **42**, 387–390.

Gan, T.J., Sloan, F., de L Dear, G., Lubarsky, D.A., El Moalem, H.E. (2001). How much are patients willing to pay to avoid postoperative nausea and vomiting? *Anesthesia and Analgesia* **92**, 393–400.

Gan, T.J. (2002). Postoperative nausea and vomiting – Can it be eliminated? *Journal of the American Medical Association* **287**, 1233–1236.

Gray, J.A.M., Haynes, R.B., Sackett, D.L., Cook, D.J., Guyatt, G.H. (1997). Transferring evidence from health care research into medical practice. 3. Developing evidence-based clinical policy. *Evidence-Based Medicine* **2**, 36–38.

Grol, R., Grimshaw, J. (1999). Evidence-based implementation of evidence-based medicine. *Journal of Quality Improvement* **25**, 503–513.

Hadji, F., Eastowood, D., Fear, S., Corfield, H.J. (1998). The impact of audit in a district general hospital on post-operative nausea and vomiting after major gynaecological surgery. *European Journal of Anaesthesiology* **15**, 595–595.

Harmer, M. (1998). The challenge of post-operative nausea and vomiting. Glaxo Wellcome UK, Uxbridge.

Harmer, M., Davies, K.A. (1998). The effect of education, assessment and a standardised prescription on postoperative pain management. The value of clinical audit in the establishment of acute pain services. *Anaesthesia* **53**, 424–430.

Hawthorn, J. (1995). Understanding and management of nausea and vomiting. Blackwell Science, Oxford.

Haynes, B., Haines, A. (1998). Barriers and bridges to evidence based clinical practice. *British Medical Journal* **317**, 273–276.

Heffernan, A.M., Rowbotham, D.J. (2000). Postoperative nausea and vomiting (Editorial). *British Journal of Anaesthesia* **85**, 675–677.

Henzi, I., Sonderegger, J., Tramer, M.R. (2000). Efficacy, dose-response and adverse effects of droperidol for prevention of postoperative nausea and vomiting. *Canadian Journal of Anaesthesia* **47**, 537–551.

Hopkins, A. (1995). Some reservations about clinical guidelines. *Archives of Disease in Childhood* **72**, 70–75.

Humphris, D. (1994). *The Clinical Nurse Specialist: Issues in Practice.* MacMillan Press, Basingstoke.

Jackson, R., Feder, G. (1998). Editorial. Guidelines for clinical guidelines. *British Medical Journal* **317**, 427–428.

Jeffrey, K.M., Harkins, B., Cresci, G.A., Martindale, R.G. (1996). The clear liquid diet is no longer a necessity in the routine postoperative management of surgical patients. *The American Surgeon* **62**, 167–171.

Jolley, S. (2000a). Patient information on post-operative sickness. *Nursing Standard* **14**, 32–34.

Jolley, S. (2000b). Post-operative nausea and vomiting: a survey of nurses' knowledge. *Nursing Standard* **14**, 32–34.

Koivuranta, M., Läärä, E., Snåre, L., Alahuhta, S. (1997). A survey of postoperative nausea and vomiting. *Anaesthesia* **52**, 443–449.

Kovac, A.L. (2000). Prevention and treatment of postoperative and vomiting. *Drugs* **59**, 213–243.

Mann, T. (1996). Clinical guidelines: using clinical guidelines to improve patient care within the NHS. Leeds: NHS Executive.

Mckenzie, R., Uy, N.T.L., Riley, T.J., Hamilton, D.L. (1996). Droperidol/ondansetron combination controls nausea and vomiting after tubal banding. *Anesthesia and Analgesia* **83**, 1218–1222.

McNicol, M., Layton, A., Morgan, G. (1993). Team working: the key to implementing guidelines? *Quality in Health Care* **2**, 215–6.

NHS Centre for Reviews and Dissemination (1999). Getting evidence into practice. *Effective Health Care* **5**, 1–16.

Nightingale, K. (1994). Postoperative nausea and vomiting. Achieving quality of care. A guide for nurses. Direct Publishing Solutions. Glaxo Laboratories Limited.

Nolte, M.J., Berkery, R., Pizzo, B. *et al.* (1998). Assuring the optimal use of serotonin antagonist anti-emetics: the process for development and implementation of institutional anti-emetic guidelines at Memorial Sloan-Kettering Cancer Center. *Journal of Clinical Oncology* **16**, 771–778.

Paech, M.J., Pavy, T.J., Kristensen, J.H., Wojnar-Horton, R.E. (1998). Postoperative nausea and vomiting: development of a management protocol. *Anaesthesia and Intensive Care* **26**, 152–155.

Royal College of Anaesthetists (2000). *Raising the standard.* London: Royal College of Anaesthetists.

Rubin, G.L., Frommer, M.S., Vincent, N.C., Phillips, P.A., Leeder, S.R. (2000). Getting new evidence into medicine. *Medical Journal of Australia* **172**, 180–183.

Scuderi, P.E., James, R.L., Harris, L., Mirns III, G.R. (2000). Multimodal anti-emetic management prevents early postoperative vomiting after outpatient laparoscopy. *Anesthesia and Analgesia* **91**, 1408–1414.

Shapiro, D.W., Lasker, R.D., Bindman, A.B., Lee, P.R. (1993). Containing costs while improving the quality of care: the role of profiling and practice guidelines. *Annual Reviews in Public Health* **14**, 219–241.

Stockdale, A., Bellman, M. (1998). An audit of post-operative pain and nausea in day case surgery. *European Journal of Anaesthesiology* **15**, 271–274.

Tate, S., Cook, S. (1996). Post-operative nausea and vomiting I; physiology and aetiology. *British Journal of Nursing* **5**, 962–973.

Thompson, H.J. (1999). The management of post-operative nausea and vomiting. *Journal of Advanced Nursing* **29**, 1130–1136.

Tramér, M., Moore, A., McQuay, H. (1997a). Meta-analytic comparison of prophylactic anti-emetic efficacy for postoperative nausea and vomiting: propofol anaesthesia vs omitting nitrous oxide vs total i.v. anaesthesia with propofol. *British Journal of Anaesthesia* **78**, 256–259.

Tramér, M.R., Moore, R.A., Reynolds, D.J.M., McQuay, H.J. (1997b). A quantitative systematic review of ondansetron in the treatment of established postoperative nausea and vomiting. *British Medical Journal* **314**, 1088–1092.

Tramér, M.R., Philips, C., Reynolds, D.J.M., Moore, R.A., McQuay, H.J. (1999). Cost-effectiveness of ondansetron for postoperative nausea and vomiting. *Anaesthesia* **54**, 226–235.

Tramer, M.R. (2000). Systematic reviews in PONV therapy. In: MR Tramer, ed. Evidence Based Resource in Anaesthesia and Analgesia. London: BMJ Books.

Tramér, M.R. (2001a). A rational approach to the control of postoperative nausea and vomiting: evidence from systematic reviews. Part I. Efficacy and harm of antiemetic interventions, and methodological issues. *Acta Anaesthesiologica Scandanavica* **45**, 4–13.

Tramér, M.R. (2001b). A rational approach to the control of postoperative nausea and vomiting: evidence from systematic reviews. Part II. Recommendations for prevention and treatment, and research agenda. *Acta Anaesthesiologica Scandanavica* **45**, 14–19.

Tsui, S.L., Irwin, M.G., Wong Fung, S.K., Hui, T.W., Ng, K.F., Chan, W.S., O'Reagan, A.M. (1997). An audit of the safety of an acute pain service. *Anaesthesia* **52**, 1042–1047.

Waterman, H., Leatherbarrow, B., Slater, R. & Waterman, C. (1999). Post-operative pain, nausea and vomiting: qualitative perspectives from telephone interviews. *Journal of Advanced Nursing* **29**, 690–696.

West, E., Newton, J. (1997). Clinical guidelines. Editorial. *British Medical Journal* **315**, 324.

Wilder-Smith, O.H.G., Martin, N.C., Morabia, A. (1997). Postoperative nausea and vomiting: a comparative survey of the attitudes, perceptions, and practice of Swiss anesthesiologists and surgeons. *Anesthesia and Analgesia* **84**, 826–831.

PART 4

Ongoing research in PONV

Chapter 9

Future research strategies for the prevention and treatment of post-operative nausea and vomiting

Phil M. Hopkins

Introduction

Post-operative nausea and vomiting (PONV) is recognised as a most distressing complication. It ranks alongside pain as the post-operative complication most feared by patients awaiting surgery. As well as being distressing for the patient, PONV delays discharge, increases nursing workload and is costly (Sanchez *et al.* 1995). An incidence of up to 90% in some surgical groups (Morris *et al.* 1998) should dictate that research into the prevention and treatment of PONV is a top priority.

There are indeed numerous reports in the anaesthetic literature of studies in the field. The area of the brain responsible for the initiation of the vomiting reflex, known as the vomiting or emetic centre, has been located to the reticular formation of the medulla (Andrews 1992). Efferent activity emanating from the vomiting centre is thought to arise in response to nociceptive afferent activity, especially that arising from abdominal and pelvic viscera. Vestibular activity is a well-known precursor of vomiting (motion sickness) as are intense emotional or psychological stimuli (Palazzo & Strunin 1984). Another region of the medulla, known as the chemoreceptor trigger zone (Borison 1989), contains a variety of receptors (Atweh & Kuhar 1977; Palacios *et al.* 1981; Wamsley *et al.* 1981; Waeber *et al.* 1988) that, when stimulated, lead to increased output from the vomiting centre. The transduction of the chemical stimulus into vomiting centre output may involve dopaminergic, cholinergic, histaminergic, serotinergic and opioid receptors, either singly or in combination. Antagonism of these receptors remains the principal pharmacological approach to the treatment and prevention of PONV (Peroutka 1982). And yet, the most successful clinical trials of any of the antagonists fail to reduce the incidence of PONV by much more than 50% (see, for example, Morris *et al.* 1998). This contrasts with the situation in the prevention and treatment of cancer chemotherapy-induced nausea and vomiting, where 5-HT_3 antagonists, such as ondansetron and granisetron, have had a huge impact (Cubeddu *et al.* 1990; Kidgell *et al.* 1990; Pintens 1990). Such a difference between the two situations indicates that additional factors may be operating in PONV, as compared with chemotherapy emesis. Indeed, cohort studies and retrospective analyses have identified several factors that predispose to PONV (see, for example, Palazzo & Evans 1993). Other than specific drugs, these include female sex, age, obesity, history of motion sickness and nature of surgery (e.g. gynaecological operations). Although such studies may be useful for targeting those patients at greatest risk of PONV, they give few clues as to the best approach to preventing PONV. Knowledge of these factors is also important, however, in the design of clinical trials in which as many confounding variables should be controlled as is practically feasible.

But perhaps before we discuss future clinical trials in PONV research, we should consider whether our fundamental knowledge is sufficient to dispense with further basic research. The lack of efficacy of current clinical approaches, and indeed the number of different approaches *per se*, indicate to this author that we do have much to learn. In a review of limited space, such as this, it would be inappropriate to detail all the possible laboratory research angles that might be considered. Instead, three research questions that are of importance to improving the management of PONV will be discussed.

Can we distinguish the properties of anaesthetic drugs responsible for the anaesthetic effect from those responsible for PONV?

The implication in asking this question is that we can identify the cellular mechanisms of anaesthesia. Importantly, however, we know that the anaesthetic properties for some groups of anaesthetic drugs do not involve mechanisms that cause nausea and vomiting. Specifically, the intravenous anaesthetics, which probably have their major anaesthetic effect through amplification of GABA-induced chloride currents (Franks & Lieb 1994), demonstrate differing propensities for inducing PONV. Thiopentone and, especially, etomidate are emetic (Horrigan *et al.* 1983; Kestin & Dorje 1987), whereas propofol is not (de Grood *et al.* 1987; Edelist *et al.* 1987), and there is some evidence that it may even have anti-emetic properties (McCollum *et al.* 1988). The situation is different with the volatile anaesthetics. These drugs also increase inhibitory chloride currents (Franks & Lieb 1994), but the magnitude of these effects is probably insufficient to explain the complete range of their anaesthetic effects. Evidence is accumulating that the volatile anaesthetics inhibit the release of excitatory neurotransmitters (Schlame & Hemmings 1995) through actions on presynaptic calcium channels and possibly also sodium channel subtypes (Lynch & Pancrazio 1994; Winlow *et al.* 1995). It can be easily envisaged how increasing inhibitory signals and inhibiting excitatory neurotransmitters might contribute to anaesthesia. It is not so clear, however, how these mechanisms would be likely to lead to increased neuronal output by the vomiting centre. Other than a potent agonistic action at some cholinergic receptor subtypes (Raines 1994), the volatile anaesthetics have little effect at receptor subtypes identified in the chemoreceptor trigger zone. This is perhaps why the conventional antagonists at these receptors appear to have limited efficacy in PONV. Many other actions of volatile anaesthetics have been described in neuronal preparations and other cell types, and some of these could plausibly lead to increased activity in the neuronal networks that make up the vomiting centre. For example, in some types of neuron, volatile anaesthetics cause an increase in intracellular Ca^{2+} concentration (Winlow *et al.* 1995), which could lead to increased neuronal activity. Such an action might, however, have a role in the anaesthetic action of these drugs. Testing of these hypotheses requires more detailed characterisation of the types of neuron present in those central pathways responsible for emetic reflexes and their responses to anaesthetic drugs.

Can the neuronal pathway of opioid-induced vomiting be identified?

Opioids are probably the single biggest culprit in causing PONV (Dundee *et al.* 1965; Pandit & Kothary 1989). The influence of opioids is perhaps more complex than might be first considered. As well as directly stimulating emesis, opioids can, through alleviation of pain, reduce nausea and the likelihood of vomiting (Anderson & Krohg 1976). The pro-emetic effects of opioids are considered to be initiated through binding to opioid (probably μ) receptors located in the chemoreceptor trigger zone. Opioid receptor antagonism is clearly not a treatment option, as the desirable analgesic effects would be antagonised also. The logical approach, therefore, would be to interrupt the pathway downstream from opioid receptor activation. Delineation of this pathway is required.

Is there a 'final common processing pathway' for the emetic reflex?

As already suggested, much more is known about the many stimuli of emesis than the neuronal pathways involved in transduction of a stimulus to produce the emetic reflex. Postulation of the vomiting centre implies that the diverse stimuli may converge to trigger a common mechanism for emesis. If this is so, the precise location of the convergence has important consequences for the likely efficacy of therapeutic interventions (Borison 1989; Andrews 1992). If we consider the vomiting centre to be a central pattern generator (CPG) – in its simplest form, a single group of identical neurons responsible for co-ordination of a defined motor response – several possibilities for afferent and efferent connections exist. Three examples are represented in Figure 9.1. The relationship in Figure 9.1(a) presents the most attractive therapeutic potential, as a drug that either reduces activity of the interneuron or blocks the effect of its neurotransmitter on the CPG should block emesis resulting from a range of stimuli. A drug that blocks the transmitter(s) released by the CPG neurons will have a similar effect. The neural connections illustrated in Figures 9.1(b) and 9.1(c) are less amenable to intervention. A drug targeted at inhibition of the CPG neurotransmitter(s) will be efficacious in the model in Figure 9.1(b) but not that in Figure 9.1(c). The connections illustrated in Figure 9.1(c) imply that multiple neurotransmitters are involved in initiation and modulation of CPG output and a combination of drugs is likely to be required to fully inhibit emesis at this level.

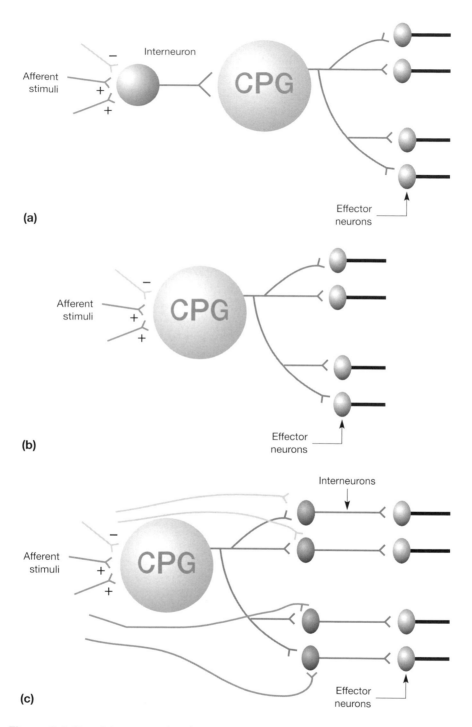

Figure 9.1 Possible neuronal pathways in the emetic reflex.

Early work using CP 99,994, a substance P antagonist acting at the neurokinin-1 (NK_1), suggested that the connections illustrated in Figures 9.1(a) and 9.1(b) may be good models for the CPG (Longmore *et al.* 1997). CP 99,994 has been shown in animal models to be effective against a wide range of stimuli, including cisplatin (5-HT and vagal stimulation), copper sulphate (gastric irritation), apomorphine (a dopamine [D2] receptor agonist) and morphine. Initial clinical studies in the setting of PONV, however, are perhaps not so encouraging as the efficacy of NK_1 receptor antagonists is by no means complete and perhaps little better than currently available drugs (Gesztes *et al.* 2000; Diemunsch *et al.* 1999). These findings are consistent with NK_1 receptor involvement in chemoreceptor trigger zone output, but not global depression of the CPG (Hornby 2001). An additional mechanism of inhibition of vagal *motor* output may make NK_1 antagonists more effective in reducing emesis than nausea (Hornby 2001).

A different approach to identify areas of the brain involved in the emetic response, which is applicable to humans, is the use of positron emission tomography. This imaging technique is able to display areas of increased neuronal activity and could be used, for example, to map activity in volunteers given emetogens.

Problems with laboratory research in PONV

The major problems arise with the suitability of animal models. A fundamental problem with some species, such as rats, rabbits and horses, is that they do not vomit. Dogs, cats and ferrets do vomit and are used in emesis research. However, it is not clear that the neuroanatomical connections involved in vomiting in these animals are sufficiently similar to that in humans for results to be extrapolated to humans. Animals that do vomit may respond in different ways to emetogenic stimuli compared to humans. For example, humans and dogs readily vomit when given apomorphine, whereas cats do not. It is also clearly impossible to use animals to study nausea as this is a subjective phenomenon.

Problems with PONV research in the clinical setting

Vomiting is an explicit end-point and it should be relatively easy to record the number of events. The subjectivity of nausea, however, means that comparisons between patients and especially between studies is more difficult. Verbal rating scales and visual analogue scores can be used to obtain a measure of severity of nausea, while some investigators prefer not to attempt to quantify the severity of nausea but rather record its duration.

Many studies of PONV have failed to contribute meaningful data because they lack sufficient statistical power (Watcha & White 1992). In this sense, the power of a study is the likelihood that the study will detect a difference of defined magnitude when that difference truly exists in the population. A study will lack power if too few patients or subjects are included in the sample. Determination of sample size is a key element of study design and appropriate expertise must be sought at this stage. A power calculation requires estimates of both the incidence of an event under study and the variability of any measure. A pilot study is often required to provide these estimates.

The presence of confounding variables complicates power calculations. With regard to PONV, I have already mentioned some confounding variables that have been shown to have an influence (e.g. age, sex, history of motion sickness, type of surgery, etc.) Good study design aims to limit the influence of confounding variables, first by appropriate inclusion and exclusion criteria and second by randomised allocation to treatment and control groups.

Strategies for limiting PONV

Three main approaches to limiting PONV can be defined:

- avoiding emetogenic stimuli;
- prophylaxis;
- treatment of established PONV.

Each of these approaches warrants further clinical research.

Reducing emetogenic stimuli

Specific triggers of PONV have been mentioned previously but there are some interesting research questions awaiting definitive study. Some illustrative cases are now considered.

The use of nitrous oxide

Several trials have investigated the influence of nitrous oxide on PONV (Lonie & Harper 1986; Korttila et al. 1987; Muir et al. 1987). The conclusions are conflicting but many of the studies are inadequately powered and do not consider confounding variables (see above). Two groups have undertaken systematic reviews in the form of meta-analyses of relevant randomised controlled trials (RCTs) (Divatia et al. 1996; Tramer et al. 1996). Both reviews were based on a similar data set, i.e. the RCTs analysed were by and large the same in both papers, but the two sets of authors drew opposite conclusions. Divatia et al. found that PONV was reduced when the use of nitrous oxide was avoided and recommended it not be used. Tramer et al., although they found an increased risk of PONV with nitrous oxide, recommended that it should be used because in a subset of the RCTs there was an unacceptably high incidence of recall of intra-operative awareness in those patients not given nitrous oxide. This is an interesting finding, but the incidence of awareness does seem extraordinarily high. I would suggest that it is perfectly possible to ensure lack of awareness while not using nitrous oxide and would offer the possible explanation that some investigators may have subconsciously attempted to deliver less anaesthetic in order to limit PONV. The important question of the benefits or otherwise of nitrous oxide needs to be addressed in a well-designed RCT.

Choice of anaesthetic drugs

There are fairly consistent data that indicate some anaesthetics are more likely to be associated with PONV. For example, etomidate is associated with a higher incidence than thiopentone, which in turn appears to be more emetogenic than propofol (Horrigan *et al.* 1983; de Grood *et al.* 1987; Edelist 1987). It has not been defined, however, in what situations these statistical differences are likely to be clinically important. It may well be, for example, that propofol is advantageous when used as a sole anaesthetic with no, or a short-acting, opioid for surgical procedures of limited duration. But this may not be the case when the intravenous anaesthetic is used only for induction of a prolonged anaesthetic, which is followed by the use of patient-controlled analgesia with morphine. This is an example of the extent of the detail required if evidence-based clinical decision making is to improve patient care.

Optimising analgesia

There is a complex relationship between pain, analgesic drugs and PONV. The aim of management is to minimise pain, which itself is associated with nausea and vomiting (Anderson & Krohg 1976), and to limit the emetogenic effects of analgesic drugs. Much can be achieved with methods of analgesia other than systemically administered opioids as these are the main culprit for causing PONV (Dundee *et al.* 1965; Pandit & Kothari 1989). In many circumstances, opioids are the best means of treating post-operative pain and here the goals can be defined as, first, can we limit the severity of pain (e.g. by using 'pre-emptive' analgesia), and second, is there a least emetogenic method of administering opioids (e.g. by optimising patient-contolled analgesia machine settings)?

Peri-operative fluid therapy

In many countries, but not the UK, an intravenous infusion during anaesthesia is a standard of care. Small prospective studies have suggested that intra-operative fluid therapy reduces the incidence of PONV. These findings need to be verified on a larger scale. Furthermore, the optimal fluid regimen needs to be determined.

Timing of pre- and post-operative oral intake

The level of evidence here is almost at the anecdotal level. It does seem plausible to suppose that either excessive or inadequate periods of pre-operative starvation might predispose to PONV. Similarly, the timing of initial fluid and food intake post-operatively is likely to be important (van den Berg *et al.* 1987).

With each of these potential emetogenic stimuli there are other considerations for the clinician. The use of any drug or technique is associated with benefits in addition to unwanted effects. The use of nitrous oxide, discussed above, is a good example. It is important that clinical trials are designed to address wanted and unwanted effects.

Pharmacological approaches to the prevention and treatment of PONV

Although it is to be hoped that new drugs will emerge from basic research to become clinically available, there are still many unanswered questions about the use of currently available anti-emetics for the indication of PONV. Some of these questions arise because the drug was not originally licensed for this indication. Droperidol, for example, was marketed originally as a neuroleptic adjunct to anaesthesia. Some efficacy in PONV was demonstrated, but so were side-effects that are occasionally distressing. Similar considerations apply to cyclizine and metoclopramide. The more recently introduced 5-HT$_3$ antagonists have been better characterised.

Specific efficacy of individual drugs

PONV is frequently considered as a single entity. There may be some benefit in attempting to identify specific triggers and, from there go on to determine the efficacy of individual drugs with respect to those specific triggers. We know that opioids, anaesthetics and visceral stimuli all cause PONV, but why should they do so by the same mechanism and, therefore, why should PONV due to each cause be equally amenable to treatment by the same drug or group of drugs? A series of carefully designed and controlled clinical trials would be needed to progress in this area.

Drug combinations

We have discussed the complex neuropharmacology of nausea and vomiting. Lack of complete efficacy of all the currently available treatments for PONV implies that either multiple receptor types, or as-yet-unidentified receptors, are involved in the production of PONV. The former hypothesis may be addressed by studying combinations of drugs that act at different receptors. If these studies are designed to include a formal evaluation of synergism, important new information about the neurophysiology of vomiting may be obtained.

Implementation of clinical research

An extensive series of RCTs would be required to address the research questions discussed above. Experimental design will be crucial. Many of the designs will require large sample sizes, and some of the study groups will have restrictive inclusion criteria. It is inevitable that adequate recruitment will demand multi-centre involvement.

Evaluation of new treatment strategies arising from research

The aim of the research described is to accumulate sufficient data to provide a detailed evidence base which will advise the formulation of treatment strategies both to prevent and treat PONV. Once designed, these treatment strategies will require prospective evaluation and audit. Included in this evaluation should be health economic analysis.

References

Anderson, R. & Krohg, K. (1976). Pain as a major cause of postoperative nausea. *Journal of the Canadian Anaesthesia Society* **23**, 366–369.

Andrews, P.L.R. (1992). Physiology of nausea and vomiting. *British Journal of Anaesthesia* **69**(Suppl.1), 2–19.

Atweh, S.F. & Kuhar, M.J. (1977). Autoradiographic localization of opiate receptors in the brain: II the brain stem. *Brain Research* **129**, 1–12.

Borison, H.L. (1989). Area postrema: chemoreceptor circumventricular organ of the medulla oblongata. *Progress in Neurobiology* **32**, 351–390.

Cubeddu, L.X., Hoffman, I.S., Fuenmayor, N.T. & Finn, A.L. (1990). Efficacy of ondansetron (GR 38032F) and the role of cisplatin-induced nausea and vomiting. *New England Journal of Medicine* **322**, 810–816.

de Grood, P.M.R.M., Mitsukuri, S., van Egmond, J., Rutten, R.M.J. & Crul, J.F. (1987). Comparison of etomidate and propofol for anaesthesia in microlaryngeal surgery. *Anaesthesia* **42**, 366–372.

Diemunsch, P., Schoeffler, P., Bryssini, B., Cheli-Muller, L.E., Lees, J., McQuade, B.A. & Spraggs, C.F. (1999). Antiemetic activity of the NK1 receptor antagonist GR205171 in the treatment of established postoperative nausea and vomiting after major gynaecological surgery. *British Journal of Anaesthesia* **82**, 274–276.

Divatia, J.V., Vaidya, J.S., Badwe, R.A. & Hawaldar, R.W. (1996). Omission of nitrous oxide during anesthesia reduces the incidence of postoperative nausea and vomiting: a meta-analysis. *Anesthesiology* **85**, 1055–1062.

Dundee, J.W., Kirwan, M.K. & Clarke, R.S.J. (1965). Anaesthesia and premedication as factors in postoperative vomiting. *Acta Anaesthesiologica Scandinavica* **9**, 223–231.

Edelist, G. (1987). A comparison of propofol and thiopentone as induction agents in outpatient surgery. *Canadian Journal of Anaesthesia* **34**, 110–116.

Franks, N.P. & Lieb, W.R. (1994). Molecular and cellular mechanisms of general anaesthesia. *Nature* **367**, 607–614.

Gesztes, Z., Sanderi, P.E., White, P.F., Wright, W., Wender, R.H., D'Angelo, R., Black, L.S., Dalby, P.L., MacLean, D. (2000). Substance P (Neurokinin-1) antagonist prevents postoperative vomiting after abdominal hysterectomy procedures. *Anaesthesiology* **93**, 931–937.

Hornby, P.J. (2001). Central neurocircuitry associated with emesis. *American Journal of Medicine* **111**(Suppl.8A), 1065–1125.

Horrigan, R.W., Moyers, J.R., Johnson, B.H., Eger, E.I. II, Margolis, A. & Goldsmith, S. (1983). Etomidate versus thiopental with and without fentanyl. A comparative study of awakening in man. *Anesthesiology* **59**, 564–569.

Kestin, I.G. & Dorje, P. (1987). Anaesthesia for evacuation of retained products of conception: comparison between alfentanil plus etomidate and fentanyl plus thiopentone. *British Journal of Anaesthesia* **59**, 364–368.

Kidgell, A.E., Butcher, M.E. & Brown, G.W. (1990). Antiemetic control: 5-HT$_3$ antagonists. Review of clinical results, with particular emphasis on ondansetron. *Cancer Treatment Reviews* **17**, 311–317.

Korttila, K., Hovorka, J. & Erkola, O. (1987). Nitrous oxide does not increase the incidence of nausea and vomiting after isoflurane anesthesia. *Anesthesia and Analgesia* **66**, 761–765.

Longmore, J., Hill, R.G. & Hargreaves, R.J. (1997). Neurokinin-receptor antagonists: pharmacological tools and therapeutic drugs. *Canadian Journal of Physiology and Pharmacology* **75**, 612–621.

Lonie, D.S. & Harper, N.J.N. (1986). Nitrous oxide and vomiting. The effect of nitrous oxide on the incidence of vomiting following gynaecological laparoscopy. *Anaesthesia* **141**, 703–707.

Lynch, C. III & Pancrazio, J.J. (1994). Snails, spiders and stereo specificity – is there a role for calcium channels in anesthetic mechanisms? *Anesthesiology* **81**, 1–5.

McCollum, J.S.C., Milligan, K.R. & Dundee, J.W. (1988). The antiemetic effect of propofol. *Anaesthesia* **43**, 239–240.

Morris, R.W., Aune, H., Feiss, P., Hanson, A., Hasselstrom, L., Maltby, J.R., Rocke, D.A., Rozenberg, B., Rust, M. & Cohen, L.A. (1998). International, multicentre, placebo-controlled study to evaluate the effectiveness of ondansetron vs. metoclopramide in the prevention of post-operative nausea and vomiting. *European Journal of Anesthesiology* **15**, 69–79.

Muir, J.J., Warner, M.A., Offord, K.J., Buck, C.F., Harper, J.V. & Kunkel, J.E. (1987). Role of nitrous oxide and other factors in nausea and vomiting. A randomized and blinded prospective study. *Anesthesiology* **66**, 513–518.

Palacios, J.M., Wamsley, J.K. & Kuhar, M.J. (1981). The distribution of H1-receptors in the rat brain: an autoradiographic study. *Neuroscience* **6**, 15–17.

Palazzo, M. & Evans, R. (1993). Logistic regression analysis of fixed patient factors for postoperative sickness: a model for risk assessment. *British Journal of Anaesthesia* **70**, 135–140.

Palazzo, M.G.A. & Strunin, L. (1984). Anaesthesia and emesis: 1. Etiology. *Journal of the Canadian Anaesthesia Society* **31**, 178–187.

Pandit, S.K. & Kothary, S.P. (1989). Intravenous narcotics for premedication in outpatient anaesthesia. *Acta Anaesthesiologica Scandinavica* **33**, 353–358.

Peroutka, S.J. & Snyder, S.H. (1982). Antiemetics: neurotransmitter receptor binding predicts therapeutic action. *Lancet* **1**, 714–716.

Pintens, H. (1990). Granisetron (BRL 43694) in the treatment of cytostatic drug-induced emesis: a summary. *Cancer Treatment Reviews* **17**, 307–310.

Raines, D.E. (1996). Anesthetic and nonanesthetic halogenated volatile compounds have dissimilar activities on nicotinic acetylcholine receptor desensitization kinetics. *Anesthesiology* **84**, 663–671.

Sanchez, L.A., Hirsch, J.D., Carroll, N.V. & Miederhoff, P.A. (1995). Estimation of the cost of postoperative nausea and vomiting in an ambulatory surgery center. *Journal of Research in Pharmacological Economics* **6**, 35–44.

Schlame, M. & Hemmings, H.C. Jr (1995). Inhibition by volatile anesthetics of endogenous glutamate release from synaptosomes by a presynaptic mechanism. *Anesthesiology* **82**, 1406–1416.

Tramer, M., Moore, A. & McQuay, H. (1996). Omitting nitrous oxide in general anaesthesia: meta-analysis of intraoperative awareness and postoperative emesis in randomized controlled trials. *British Journal of Anaesthesia* **76**, 186–193.

van den Berg, A.A., Lambourne, A., Yazji, N.S., Laghari, N.A. *et al.* (1987). Vomiting after ophthalmic surgery: effects of intraoperative antiemetics and postoperative oral fluid restriction. *Anaesthesia* **42**, 270–276.

Waeber, C., Dixon, K., Hoyer, D. & Palacios, J.M. (1988). Localisation by autoradiography of neuronal 5-HT$_3$ receptors in the mouse. *European Journal of Pharmacology* **151**, 351–352.

Wamsley, J.K., Lewis, M.S., Young, W.S. III & Kuhar, M.J. (1981). Autoradiographic localization of muscarinic cholinergic receptors in rat brainstem. *Journal of Neurosciece* **1**, 176–191

Watcha, M.F. & White, P.F. (1992). Postoperative nausea and vomiting: its etiology, treatment and prevention. *Anesthesiology* **77**, 162–184.

Winlow, W., Hopkins, P.M., Moghadam, H.F., Ahmed, I.A. & Yar, T. (1995). Multiple cellular and subcellular actions of general anaesthetics on cultured molluscan neurones. *Acta Biologica Hungarica* **46**, 381–393.

Index

Throughout this index, the abbreviation PONV is used for post-operative nausea and vomiting.